Trauma-Informed Midwifery Care

The Essential Handbook for Practice, Protocols, and Provider Resilience

May Ivette Ray

Table of Contents

Chapter 1: The Reality of Trauma in the Perinatal Period

You went into midwifery because you wanted to make a difference. You wanted to support people during one of the most vulnerable times in their lives. You pictured partnership, respect, and healthy births.

Then you started practicing.

You met the client who wouldn't let you touch her, even for a simple blood pressure check. You saw the person in labor who seemed to just disappear behind their eyes—completely unreachable—while the monitors beeped steadily. You dealt with the postpartum client who seemed angry, hostile, and resistant to every piece of advice you offered.

It's frustrating, right? You might have thought, "Why are they acting like this? If they would just listen, this would be so much easier."

Here's the hard truth: The problem often isn't them. The problem is that the standard model of maternity care is built on a faulty assumption. It assumes the birthing person feels safe in medical environments. It assumes their bodies and minds haven't been shaped by terrifying experiences.

And those assumptions are often dead wrong.

When we don't understand trauma, we inevitably cause more of it. We re-traumatize the very people we are supposed to be caring for. This chapter is about facing that reality. It's about understanding what trauma actually is, how common it is, and how it shows up when people are having babies.

What We Get Wrong About Trauma

Let's clear something up right away. Trauma is not just a bad memory. It's not just feeling sad about something that happened in the past.

When we talk about psychological trauma, we are talking about a fundamental change in the nervous system.

We often think of trauma as the big, obvious events: war, natural disasters, or severe physical assault. Yes, those are traumatic. But trauma is much broader. It includes experiences of abuse, neglect, systemic oppression, and even seemingly routine medical procedures.

The most useful definition of trauma comes from the Substance Abuse and Mental Health Services Administration (SAMHSA). They break it down using the "Three E's": Event, Experience, and Effect (SAMHSA, 2014).

The Three E's

1. **The Event:** This is the thing that happened. It could be a single incident, like a car accident or a sexual assault. Or it could be chronic, like ongoing childhood neglect, living in poverty, or experiencing daily racism. The event involves a threat to physical or psychological safety.
2. **The Experience:** This is the critical part. How the individual experiences the event determines whether it is traumatic. If the person feels overwhelmed, helpless, terrified, or trapped, the event is experienced as trauma. Two people can go through the same event, but experience it completely differently. If a person feels supported and validated during a difficult event, it may not become imprinted as trauma. If they feel alone and terrified, it likely will.
3. **The Effect:** These are the long-term results of the trauma. Effects can be immediate or delayed. They include changes in the brain and body, such as chronic hyperarousal (always being on alert), difficulty regulating emotions, physical health problems, relationship issues, and mental health conditions like PTSD, depression, and anxiety.

Why does this definition matter in midwifery? Because it tells us that **we cannot judge whether an event was traumatic based on our own perception of it.**

Think about birth. You might see a birth as clinically successful—a healthy baby, a stable parent. But if the birthing person experienced that event as terrifying, degrading, or violating, it was traumatic for them.

Birth trauma is a specific type of psychological trauma that occurs during or as a result of childbirth. It's not just about the physical injuries, though those certainly contribute. It's about the psychological experience of fear, helplessness, loss of control, and lack of care (Beck, 2004).

Examples of events that can lead to birth trauma include:

- Unplanned Cesarean sections.
- Use of forceps or vacuum extraction.
- Severe perineal tearing.
- Hemorrhage.
- The baby going to the NICU.

But here's the thing that often gets missed: birth trauma is frequently caused by how the providers behave. Things like:

- Loss of autonomy and control.
- Lack of consent for procedures.
- Feeling unheard or dismissed.
- Disrespectful, coercive, or abusive language.
- Feeling abandoned or unsupported.

When a midwife performs a cervical exam without asking, or speaks dismissively about a patient's pain, they are creating an event that is likely to be experienced as traumatic.

The 45% Reality Prevalence and Statistics

You might be thinking, "Okay, I get it. Trauma happens. But how common is it really? Surely most of my clients are fine."

Let's look at the numbers. They are staggering.

Research consistently shows that a significant portion of the population has a history of trauma. The Adverse Childhood Experiences (ACEs) study, a landmark investigation by the CDC and Kaiser Permanente, found that nearly two-thirds of adults have experienced at least one ACE (Felitti et al., 1998). ACEs include things like physical, emotional, or sexual abuse; neglect; parental mental illness; substance abuse; incarceration; divorce; and domestic violence.

Now, let's focus on the perinatal period.

- **Birth Trauma:** Studies vary, but the consensus is alarming. Up to **45% of birthing people report that their birth was traumatic** (Creedy et al., 2000; Harris & Ayers, 2012). That's nearly half of the people you care for.
- **Postpartum PTSD:** As a result of traumatic births, between 3% and 16% of women develop Post-Traumatic Stress Disorder (PTSD) postpartum (Yildiz et al., 2017). For those with previous trauma histories, the rates are even higher.

Let that sink in. If you see 10 clients, 4 or 5 of them may perceive their birth experience as traumatic. And many more are coming into your care with existing trauma histories that will be reactivated during the perinatal period.

Consider Sarah, a 28-year-old pregnant with her first child. She comes to her prenatal appointments seeming quiet and withdrawn. She flinches when the doppler gel is cold and avoids eye contact. When the midwife discusses the upcoming glucose test, Sarah gets agitated and says she doesn't want to do it. The midwife, rushed and tired, tells her it's mandatory and she needs to cooperate for the baby's sake.

What the midwife doesn't know is that Sarah has a history of childhood medical trauma. The clinical environment, the lack of control, and the feeling of being coerced are all triggering her trauma response. By pushing her, the midwife is confirming Sarah's deeply held belief that medical providers are unsafe.

The statistics are not just numbers. They are the people sitting in your waiting room. Trauma is the norm, not the exception. Therefore, our care must be trauma-informed by default.

Types of Trauma Impacting Birth

The perinatal period is a time of intense vulnerability. The physical changes, the hormonal shifts, and the psychological transition to parenthood can all reactivate past trauma. It's like the volume gets turned up on everything.

Understanding the types of trauma your clients may have experienced is essential for providing safe and effective care.

Sexual Abuse and Assault

This is a major one. Statistics show that 1 in 4 women and 1 in 6 men have experienced sexual abuse in their lifetime (Black et al., 2011). For these survivors, pregnancy and birth can be minefields.

Think about what standard maternity care involves: intimate exams, exposure of genitals, being touched by strangers, pressure in the pelvic area, and a feeling of loss of control. These are all potent triggers for sexual abuse survivors.

A cervical exam, which you might view as a routine clinical procedure, can feel like a violation to a survivor. The sensations of labor—the intensity, the pain, the feeling of the body opening—can trigger flashbacks of the abuse.

When a survivor is triggered, they may fight back, freeze, or dissociate (we'll talk more about these responses in Chapter 2). They are not trying to be difficult. Their body is responding to a perceived threat based on past experiences.

Medical Trauma

Many people have experienced trauma within the healthcare system. This can stem from childhood experiences, life-saving but terrifying interventions, chronic illness management, or previous disrespectful care.

Medical trauma is the psychological response to stressful medical experiences. It can look like:

- Fear of hospitals or clinics.
- Distrust of medical providers.
- Avoiding necessary care.
- Extreme anxiety during procedures.

If a person has a history of medical trauma, pregnancy and birth—which involve constant interaction with the healthcare system—will be incredibly challenging. They may seem hyper-vigilant, asking excessive questions, or conversely, completely shut down and passive.

Intimate Partner Violence (IPV)

Intimate partner violence (IPV), which includes physical, sexual, emotional, and financial abuse, is tragically common. Pregnancy can be a particularly dangerous time, as abuse often escalates during this period (Silverman et al., 2006).

IPV survivors are dealing with ongoing trauma and safety concerns. They may miss appointments, have inconsistent explanations for injuries, or have a partner who is overly controlling and refuses to leave the room.

Providing trauma-informed care for IPV survivors involves recognizing the signs, asking sensitive questions in private, ensuring confidentiality, and providing resources and safety planning. The primary goal is safety—both physical and psychological.

Systemic Oppression and Racial Trauma

This is a type of trauma that is often ignored in healthcare education, but it is pervasive and significantly impacts birth outcomes.

Systemic oppression refers to the ways in which society is structured to benefit dominant groups while disadvantaging marginalized groups. This includes racism, sexism, homophobia, transphobia, ableism, and poverty.

Racial trauma is the mental and emotional injury caused by encounters with racial bias and discrimination, racism, and hate crimes (Comas-Díaz, 2016).

For Black, Indigenous, and other People of Color (BIPOC), interacting with the healthcare system is inherently stressful. There is a long history of medical abuse and exploitation of BIPOC communities, leading to a deep-seated distrust of providers.

We see the effects of this trauma in the appalling disparities in maternal mortality rates. In the United States, Black women are three to four times more likely to die from pregnancy-related causes than white women (CDC, 2020). This is not due to biology. It is due to racism and bias in the healthcare system.

BIPOC clients may come into your care expecting to be mistreated, dismissed, or harmed. They may be hyper-vigilant, needing to advocate fiercely for themselves, or they may be shut down as a protective mechanism.

Trauma-informed care requires recognizing the reality of racial trauma and actively working to provide culturally safe and anti-racist care. It means believing BIPOC clients when they say they are in pain. It means addressing your own biases and understanding how they impact your practice.

Intergenerational Trauma

Trauma doesn't just disappear when the person who experienced it dies. It can be passed down through generations.

Intergenerational trauma is the transmission of the emotional and behavioral effects of trauma from one generation to the next (Yehuda & Lehrner, 2018). This can happen through parenting styles, attachment patterns, cultural narratives, and even biological changes (epigenetics).

For example, descendants of Holocaust survivors, or Indigenous people whose ancestors survived genocide and forced relocation, carry the imprint of that trauma in their nervous systems. They may have higher levels of stress hormones, increased anxiety, and a heightened sensitivity to threat.

When caring for clients from communities with histories of collective trauma, it's important to understand this context. Their responses to stress and their needs for safety may be shaped by experiences they didn't personally live through, but which live on within them.

The Long-Term Impact on Bonding Feeding and Mental Health

Trauma during the perinatal period doesn't end when the birth is over. It has lasting effects on the parent, the baby, and the family unit. When we fail to provide trauma-informed care, we contribute to these negative outcomes.

Impact on Bonding and Attachment

The immediate postpartum period is a critical time for bonding between the parent and the baby. When a parent has experienced a traumatic birth, this process can be severely disrupted.

If the parent is struggling with PTSD symptoms—flashbacks, nightmares, emotional numbness, or irritability—they may find it difficult to connect with their baby. They may feel detached, resentful, or even fearful of the baby, who serves as a constant reminder of the trauma (Beck & Watson, 2008).

A trauma survivor's nervous system is often stuck in a state of high alert. This makes it hard to be present, attuned, and responsive to the baby's needs—all of which are essential for secure attachment. The baby, sensing the parent's stress and disconnection, may become fussy, difficult to soothe, or withdrawn, creating a negative feedback loop.

Consider Maria, who had an emergency Cesarean section after a long and terrifying labor. She felt helpless and violated during the procedure. Now, at home, she struggles to hold her baby. She feels numb and disconnected. When the baby cries, she feels a surge of panic and anger. She thinks she's a terrible mother, which further compounds her distress.

Impact on Feeding

Infant feeding, whether breastfeeding/chestfeeding or bottle-feeding, is often a major challenge for trauma survivors.

For sexual abuse survivors, breastfeeding can be triggering. The physical sensation, the feeling of being needed and touched constantly, can feel overwhelming or repulsive. They may experience pain, anxiety, or dissociation during feeding.

A traumatic birth can also interfere with the physiological processes of lactation. High levels of stress hormones (like cortisol) can delay milk production and inhibit the let-down reflex (Kendall-Tackett, 2007).

Providers who are not trauma-informed may pressure survivors to breastfeed, using judgmental language like "breast is best," without understanding the underlying reasons for their struggles. This can cause further distress and shame.

Trauma-informed feeding support means respecting the parent's choices, validating their experiences, and offering practical strategies to make feeding feel safe and manageable.

Impact on Mental Health

The link between trauma and perinatal mental health conditions is undeniable. A history of trauma significantly increases the risk of developing postpartum depression (PPD), anxiety (PPA), and PTSD.

A traumatic birth experience is a major risk factor for PPD (Ayers et al., 2016). When a person feels unsupported, dismissed, or violated during birth, they are more likely to experience feelings of sadness, hopelessness, and worthlessness postpartum.

It's important to recognize that the symptoms of trauma can overlap with PPD and PPA, making diagnosis difficult. A trauma survivor may be irritable, anxious, and have trouble sleeping. But the root cause is the trauma, and the treatment needs to address that.

Furthermore, the shame and guilt associated with trauma can prevent people from seeking help. They may feel like they failed at birth, or that they are broken.

Shifting Our Viewpoint

Understanding the scope of trauma in the perinatal period is the first step toward changing how we practice. It requires a basic shift in viewpoint.

We must move away from the biomedical model, which focuses solely on the physical aspects of birth, and embrace an approach that recognizes the interconnectedness of the mind, body, and spirit.

We must stop asking "What's wrong with you?" and start asking "What happened to you?" (And sometimes, "What is happening to you right now in this system?").

This means recognizing that the "difficult" client is likely a triggered client. The "non-compliant" client is likely a client trying to protect themselves. The "anxious" client is likely a client whose nervous system is screaming danger.

It's not easy work. It requires self-reflection, education, and a commitment to changing the culture of maternity care. But it is necessary work. Because when we understand trauma, we can create safety. And when we create safety, we can truly support the people we are privileged to care for.

In the next chapter, we'll look closer at what is actually happening in the brain and body during a trauma response, so you can recognize it when it happens and know how to respond effectively.

Key Takeaways

- Trauma is defined by the individual's experience of an event and its effects, not just the event itself (The Three E's: Event, Experience, Effect).

- Birth trauma is psychological trauma occurring during or because of childbirth, often related to loss of control, lack of consent, and disrespectful care.

- Up to 45% of birthing people report their birth as traumatic. Trauma is the norm, not the exception.

- Various types of trauma impact birth, including sexual abuse, medical trauma, intimate partner violence, systemic oppression/racial trauma, and intergenerational trauma.

- The perinatal period is a time of heightened vulnerability that can reactivate past trauma.

- Trauma during the perinatal period has long-term negative impacts on bonding, feeding, and mental health.

- A trauma-informed approach requires shifting from "What's wrong with you?" to "What happened to you?"

Chapter 2: The Neurobiology of Trauma and Birth

It's tempting to think that if you are just kind enough, you can overcome a patient's trauma history. If you use a soothing voice and offer reassurance, everything will be fine. Right?

Wrong. That belief is irrational. It assumes that trauma is just about feelings or memories. But it's not. Trauma is biology. It is wired into the brain and the nervous system.

When a patient is triggered—when they are panicking, shutting down, or becoming hostile—they are not choosing to behave this way. They are having an involuntary physiological reaction. Their body is responding to a perceived threat, even if you can't see one.

If you try to reason with someone in the middle of a trauma response, you will fail. It's like trying to argue with a fire alarm to stop ringing while the house is burning down. You have to deal with the fire first.

To provide effective care, you need to understand the mechanics of what's happening. You don't need a degree in neuroscience, but you do need a basic understanding of how the brain and the nervous system work when they sense danger. This understanding will help you recognize trauma responses when they happen and intervene in a way that actually helps, instead of making things worse.

How the Brain and Nervous System Store Trauma

Our brains are designed for survival. They are constantly scanning the environment for danger. When a threat is detected, the brain activates a survival response. This system is incredibly effective at keeping us alive. But when the threat is overwhelming or chronic, the system can get stuck in "on" mode.

Let's look at three key parts of the brain involved in the trauma response.

The Amygdala The Smoke Detector

The *amygdala* is a small structure deep inside the brain. Think of it as your brain's smoke detector. Its job is to detect danger and sound the alarm.

When the amygdala detects a threat, it triggers the release of stress hormones (like adrenaline and cortisol) that prepare the body for fight or flight. This happens instantly, before you even have time to think about it.

In trauma survivors, the amygdala is often hypersensitive. It's like a smoke detector that goes off when you burn toast. It detects danger even when there is none, based on past experiences.

In the clinical setting, a trigger could be anything that reminds the brain of the original trauma. A smell, a sound, a physical sensation, a tone of voice.

Let's say you have a patient, Alex, who was sexually assaulted in a brightly lit room. When Alex walks into the brightly lit operating room for a C-section, their amygdala might sound the alarm, even though they are currently safe.

The Hippocampus The Memory Keeper

The *hippocampus* is responsible for processing memories and putting them in context. It's like a librarian that catalogs experiences and gives them a time stamp. "This happened yesterday." "This happened ten years ago."

But during a traumatic event, the high levels of stress hormones interfere with the hippocampus's function. It goes offline. As a result, traumatic memories are not processed and stored properly. They remain fragmented—bits and pieces of images, sounds, and sensations—and they don't get a time stamp (Van der Kolk, 2014).

This is why trauma survivors experience flashbacks. When a traumatic memory is triggered, the brain doesn't recognize it as something from the past. **It feels like it is happening right now.** The person is not just remembering the trauma; they are re-experiencing it.

The Prefrontal Cortex The Thinking Brain

The *prefrontal cortex* (PFC) is the part of the brain responsible for rational thought, decision-making, emotional regulation, and language. This is the "thinking brain."

When the amygdala sounds the alarm, the PFC goes offline. This is a survival mechanism. If you are being chased by a bear, you don't want to waste time thinking about your options. You just run.

But in the clinical setting, this shutdown of the PFC means that a triggered patient cannot think clearly, process information, or communicate effectively. If you are trying to explain a procedure or get informed consent from a triggered patient, they literally cannot hear you. Their thinking brain is offline.

If you keep talking at them, demanding answers, you are just escalating the situation. You must recognize that you are dealing with a physiological event, not a behavioral choice.

The Nervous System and Polyvagal Theory

Trauma doesn't just live in the brain. It lives in the body. The nervous system is the pathway through which the brain communicates with the rest of the body.

The *autonomic nervous system* (ANS) regulates involuntary functions like heart rate, breathing, and digestion. It's also responsible for the stress response.

Dr. Stephen Porges developed the *Polyvagal Theory*, which provides a very useful framework for understanding how the nervous system responds to stress and safety (Porges, 2011).

Think of the nervous system as having three states, like a traffic light:

1. **Green: Ventral Vagal (Social Engagement).** This is the state of safety and connection. When we are in the green zone, we feel calm, regulated, and open to interacting with others. Our heart rate is steady, our breathing is relaxed. This is the ideal state for birth.
2. **Yellow: Sympathetic (Fight or Flight).** When we detect a threat, we move into the yellow zone. This is the mobilization response. The sympathetic nervous system kicks in, releasing adrenaline and cortisol. Our heart rate and blood pressure go up, our muscles tense, and we feel anxious, agitated, or angry. We are ready to fight the danger or run away from it.
3. **Red: Dorsal Vagal (Freeze or Shutdown).** If the threat is overwhelming and we cannot fight or flee, we move into the red zone. This is the immobilization response. It's the body's last resort for survival. The dorsal vagal system takes over, causing us to shut down, collapse, or dissociate. Our heart rate and blood pressure drop, we might feel numb or disconnected from our body.

Trauma survivors often spend a lot of time in the yellow or red zones. Their nervous systems are constantly primed for danger. They have difficulty finding their way back to the green zone of safety.

The Physiology of Fear Fight Flight Freeze and Fawn Responses

These nervous system states translate into specific behaviors. These are the trauma responses you will see in the clinical setting. You must stop seeing these as intentional behaviors and start seeing them as automatic survival strategies.

Fight

The fight response is about confronting the threat. In the clinical setting, this might look like:

- Anger, irritability, or aggression.

- Yelling, swearing, or arguing with providers.
- Pushing people away physically.
- Being demanding or controlling.

It's easy to label a patient in fight mode as "difficult" or "aggressive." But this is a defensive response. They are trying to protect themselves because they feel unsafe. If you respond with defensiveness or aggression, you are just confirming their belief that they are in danger.

Flight

The flight response is about escaping the threat. This might look like:

- Anxiety, panic, or restlessness.
- Trying to leave the room or the hospital.
- Avoiding appointments or procedures.
- Rapid speech or difficulty focusing.

A patient in flight mode might seem "anxious" or "scattered." They are desperately trying to get away from the perceived danger.

Freeze

The freeze response is about immobilization when fight or flight is not possible. This is very common in situations where a person feels trapped, like during a medical procedure or labor. This might look like:

- Holding their breath or shallow breathing.
- Muscular tension, rigidity, or stiffness.
- Feeling stuck or unable to move.
- Blank stare or glazed eyes.
- Difficulty speaking or responding to questions.

A patient in freeze mode might seem "checked out" or even calm. But they are not calm. They are terrified. Their nervous system is overwhelmed.

Fawn

The *fawn* response is less commonly discussed, but it is very common in healthcare settings. It involves immediately trying to please or appease the perceived threat (the provider) to avoid conflict or harm (Walker, 2013). This is often learned in childhood, especially in abusive relationships.

This might look like:

- Excessive compliance or deference to authority.
- Difficulty saying no or expressing preferences.
- Apologizing excessively.
- Ignoring their own needs or pain to keep the provider happy.

This is the trickiest response to recognize because it looks like the "perfect patient." They are compliant, agreeable, and easy to manage. But this compliance is coming from a place of fear, not genuine consent. **Compliance does not equal consent.** The person is abandoning their own needs and boundaries to feel safe. If you take advantage of this, you are causing harm.

Impact of Trauma on Hormones During Pregnancy and Labor

Birth is a hormonal process. It relies on a delicate balance of hormones working together to facilitate labor, birth, and bonding. Trauma and the resulting stress response can severely disrupt this process.

The Role of Oxytocin

Oxytocin is the hormone that drives birth. It is often called the "love hormone." It is responsible for:

- Causing uterine contractions during labor.
- Promoting feelings of calm, connection, and safety.
- Facilitating bonding and attachment after birth.
- Triggering the milk ejection reflex during lactation.

Oxytocin is released when we feel safe, loved, and supported. It thrives in environments that are warm, dark, quiet, private, and undisturbed (Buckley, 2015). Think about the conditions that promote intimacy. It's the same conditions that promote oxytocin release during birth.

The Impact of Stress Hormones (Cortisol and Adrenaline)

When a person feels threatened or unsafe, their body releases stress hormones, primarily *cortisol* and *adrenaline* (also known as epinephrine). These hormones are essential for survival in acute danger. They prepare the body for fight or flight.

But in the context of labor, these stress hormones directly interfere with the process of birth.

- **Inhibition of Oxytocin:** High levels of cortisol and adrenaline inhibit the release of oxytocin. This makes sense from an evolutionary perspective. If you are being chased by a predator, it is not a good time to give birth. Your body wants to stop labor so you can get to safety.
- **Slowing or Stalling Labor:** When oxytocin is inhibited, contractions can become less effective, slower, or even stop altogether. This is a common cause of "failure to progress." But it's not a failure of the body. It's a success of the survival mechanism.
- **Fetal Distress:** Stress hormones cross the placenta and affect the baby. High levels of adrenaline can reduce blood flow to the uterus and the baby, potentially leading to fetal distress.
- **Increased Pain Perception:** Stress and fear increase the perception of pain. When we are tense and afraid, we experience contractions as more painful. This leads to the fear-tension-pain cycle described by Dr. Grantly Dick-Read (1944).

Fear causes tension, tension causes pain, and pain causes more fear.

The Midwife's Role in the Hormonal Dance

As a midwife, one of your primary roles is to protect the physiological process of birth. This means creating an environment that promotes the release of oxytocin and minimizes the release of stress hormones.

When a patient with a trauma history is triggered during labor, their body is flooded with stress hormones. This not only causes emotional distress but also directly impacts the progress of labor and the well-being of the baby.

Consider this scenario: Jessica is a survivor of childhood sexual abuse. She is in labor and doing well in a quiet, dimly lit room with her partner and midwife. Suddenly, a new nurse walks in, flips on the bright overhead lights, and starts asking rapid-fire questions without introducing herself. Jessica immediately tenses up. Her amygdala detects a threat. Her body releases adrenaline. Her contractions, which were coming every three minutes, suddenly space out to every ten minutes.

If the midwife doesn't recognize this as a trauma response and intervene to restore safety, Jessica's labor might stall. This often leads to interventions like Pitocin augmentation, which can then lead to a cascade of other interventions, potentially ending in a traumatic birth.

Your presence, your demeanor, your voice, and the environment you create directly impact the hormonal balance of birth. You are not just a passive observer. You are an active participant in the physiological process.

Recognizing Trauma Responses in the Clinical Setting

To provide trauma-informed care, you must be able to recognize when a patient is triggered. This requires paying close attention not just to what they are saying, but also to their body language, their physiology, and the subtle cues that indicate a shift in their nervous system state.

Hyperarousal (Fight or Flight)

Hyperarousal is the state of being constantly on edge, anxious, or vigilant. It corresponds to the sympathetic state (the yellow zone). Signs of hyperarousal include:

- **Vital Signs:** Increased heart rate and blood pressure that don't match the clinical situation.
- **Breathing:** Rapid or shallow breathing. Holding their breath.
- **Muscles:** Clenched fists, tight jaws, raised shoulders, rigidity in the body.
- **Movement:** Restlessness, agitation, fidgeting, constantly shifting positions.
- **Startle Response:** Jumping at sudden noises or movements.
- **Speech and Focus:** Rapid speech, jumping from topic to topic, difficulty answering questions.
- **Emotion:** Anxiety, panic, overwhelm, fear, anger.

Dissociation and Hypoarousal (Freeze or Shutdown)

Dissociation is a disconnection from one's thoughts, feelings, memories, or sense of self. It is a spectrum, ranging from mild spacing out to complete detachment from reality. It often corresponds to the dorsal vagal state (the red zone), also known as *hypoarousal*.

Signs of dissociation and hypoarousal include:

- **Eyes:** Blank stare, glazed eyes, staring off into the distance.
- **Facial Expression:** Flat affect, blank or emotionless expression, even during painful procedures or intense contractions.
- **Body Sensation:** Reporting feeling numb, floaty, or like they are watching themselves from outside their body (*depersonalization*).

- **Speech and Response:** Trouble finding words, speaking in a monotone voice, or not responding at all to questions.
- **Memory:** Gaps in memory about the appointment or the birth.
- **Behavior:** Overly compliant (fawn response), passive, still, quiet.

Avoidance

Avoidance is the attempt to stay away from anything that reminds the person of the trauma. This can significantly impact engagement with maternity care. Signs of avoidance include:

- **Appointments:** Frequently canceling appointments or showing up late, especially for appointments involving intimate exams.
- **Procedures:** Refusing cervical checks, vaginal ultrasounds, or other procedures that feel invasive or triggering.
- **Decision-Making:** Struggling to make decisions about their care, deferring to the provider or their partner.
- **Minimizing Symptoms:** Downplaying pain or discomfort to avoid attention or intervention.
- **Coping Mechanisms:** Using alcohol or drugs to cope with distress or avoid difficult feelings.

The Importance of Context

It's important to remember that these signs can also be caused by other factors, such as pain, fatigue, or medical conditions. The key is to look for patterns and changes in behavior that seem out of context or disproportionate to the situation.

For example, it's normal to be anxious during labor. But if a patient suddenly goes from calm and engaged to panicked and unable to speak during a routine cervical check, that's a red flag for a trauma response.

Tuning In and Co-Regulation

Recognizing trauma responses requires you to be present and attuned to your patients. You can't do this if you are rushed, distracted, or focused solely on the chart or the monitor. You have to look at the person in front of you.

It also requires you to be aware of your own body and nervous system. Our nervous systems are constantly communicating with each other. This is called *co-regulation*.

If you are feeling stressed, anxious, or overwhelmed, your patient will pick up on it. Your dysregulation will trigger their dysregulation. If you walk into the room rushed and frantic, you are communicating to their nervous system that the situation is unsafe.

Conversely, if you are calm, grounded, and regulated, you can help your patient feel safer and more regulated. Your calm presence can be a powerful intervention. This means taking a deep breath before you enter the room, softening your gaze, slowing down your speech, and being mindful of your body language.

You cannot expect your patients to be regulated if you are not. Self-regulation is not a luxury; it is a prerequisite for providing trauma-informed care.

The Window of Tolerance

Another useful concept is the *Window of Tolerance* (Siegel, 1999). This is the optimal zone of arousal where a person is able to function effectively and feel calm and connected. It's the green zone.

When a person is within their window of tolerance, they can handle stress and challenges without becoming overwhelmed. They can think clearly, regulate their emotions, and connect with others.

Trauma survivors often have a very narrow window of tolerance. It doesn't take much to push them outside of their window into hyperarousal (chaos) or hypoarousal (rigidity).

Your job as a midwife is to help your clients stay within their window of tolerance, or return to it if they become dysregulated. This requires recognizing the signs of dysregulation and responding in ways that promote safety and connection.

What Happens Next

Now that you understand the neurobiology of trauma, you can see why standard maternity care practices can be so triggering and counterproductive for trauma survivors. You also have the knowledge to recognize when a trauma response is happening.

Understanding the biology is not about diagnosing or labeling people. It's about shifting your perspective. It's about moving from judgment to curiosity. When you see a patient behaving in a way that seems challenging, instead of thinking, "What's wrong with them?", you can ask yourself, "What's happening in their nervous system right now?"

In the next chapter, we'll look at the core principles of trauma-informed care. These principles provide a roadmap for changing how we practice, moving from a model that risks re-traumatization to a model that promotes safety, autonomy, and healing.

Key Takeaways

- Trauma is biology, not just psychology. Trauma responses are involuntary physiological reactions, not intentional behaviors.

- The amygdala (smoke detector) detects threats, the hippocampus (memory keeper) stores memories, and the prefrontal cortex (thinking brain) is responsible for rational thought.

- During a trauma response, the thinking brain goes offline. You cannot reason with a triggered person.

- Polyvagal Theory describes three nervous system states: Ventral Vagal (safety), Sympathetic (fight or flight), and Dorsal Vagal (freeze or shutdown).

- The main trauma responses are Fight, Flight, Freeze, and Fawn. Compliance (fawn response) does not equal consent.

- Birth relies on oxytocin, which is released when we feel safe. Stress hormones (cortisol and adrenaline) inhibit oxytocin, slow labor, and increase pain (Fear-Tension-Pain cycle).

- Recognizing trauma responses (hyperarousal, dissociation/hypoarousal, avoidance) requires paying attention to body language, physiology, and behavioral cues.

- Your own regulated presence can help your patient feel safer (co-regulation).

Chapter 3: The Core Principles of TIC in Practice

Okay, we've covered what trauma is, how common it is, and how it affects the brain and body. Now what? How do we translate this knowledge into practical action? This is where trauma-informed care (TIC) comes in.

You might be thinking, "This all sounds good in theory, but how am I supposed to do this in the real world? I'm busy. I have limited time and resources. I can't change the whole system."

I hear you. The system is broken. It's designed for efficiency, not healing. But you don't have to wait for the system to change to start practicing differently. You can start implementing TIC right now, in your own practice, one interaction at a time.

But let's be clear: TIC is not a checklist. It's not a script you follow or a form you fill out. It's a fundamental shift in how you approach your work. It's a lens through which you view every interaction, every policy, and every procedure.

The goal of TIC is twofold: first, to avoid re-traumatizing people by recognizing how the healthcare system itself can be harmful. And second, to create opportunities for healing and resilience by providing care that is based on safety, collaboration, and choice.

This chapter is about the core principles of TIC and what they actually look like in the messy reality of midwifery practice.

Shifting the Paradigm From "What's Wrong with You?" to "What Happened to You?"

The traditional medical model is focused on pathology. It asks, "What's wrong with you?" and tries to fix it. This model works well for acute medical problems. If someone has a broken leg, you want to know what's wrong and how to fix it.

But when it comes to trauma, this model fails. Trauma is not a pathology. It's an injury. And the behaviors and symptoms that result from trauma are not signs of brokenness; they are adaptations. They are the ways a person learned to survive in a dangerous world.

If a patient is refusing a cervical check, the traditional model might label them as "non-compliant" and try to convince them to agree to the procedure. The focus is on the behavior as the problem.

A trauma-informed approach shifts the focus. Instead of asking, "What's wrong with you?" we ask, "What happened to you?" (SAMHSA, 2014).

When we ask "What happened to you?", we are acknowledging that the person's behavior makes sense in the context of their life experiences. We are shifting from judgment to curiosity.

In the case of the refused cervical check, a trauma-informed midwife would recognize this as a potential trauma response. They might say something like, "It seems like this procedure is difficult for you. Can we talk about what might make it feel safer?" The focus is on understanding the underlying need for safety, not just compliance.

This shift in perspective changes everything. It changes how you talk to patients, how you document their care, and how you design your services. **It moves us from being adversaries to allies.**

Reviewing the SAMHSA Principles

The Substance Abuse and Mental Health Services Administration (SAMHSA) has identified six core principles of trauma-informed care (SAMHSA, 2014). These principles provide a framework for implementing a trauma-informed approach in any setting. Let's look at how they apply to midwifery.

1. Safety

Safety is the foundation of trauma-informed care. Without safety, nothing else matters. If the nervous system detects a threat, it will activate a survival response (fight, flight, freeze, or fawn), making it impossible for the person to engage in healing and connection.

For trauma survivors, the world often feels inherently unsafe. Their nervous systems are constantly scanning for danger.

Safety means both physical and psychological safety.

- **Physical Safety:** This means ensuring that the physical environment is safe and comfortable. Think about your clinic or birth room. Is the lighting harsh or soft? Is it noisy or calm? Are there locks on the doors? The key is to minimize environmental triggers.
- **Psychological Safety:** This is about creating an atmosphere where people feel safe to be vulnerable, express their needs, and set boundaries. It means treating everyone with respect and dignity. It means being predictable, consistent, and reliable.

In midwifery practice, prioritizing safety means:

- **Introductions:** Explaining who you are and what your role is. Every time.
- **Predictability:** Clearly communicating what to expect during appointments and procedures. No surprises.
- **Privacy:** Ensuring privacy and minimizing intrusions. Knocking before entering the room. Keeping the person covered as much as possible.
- **Boundaries:** Respecting physical boundaries and asking for permission before touching.
- **Belief:** Believing survivors when they disclose trauma or express fear.

2. Trustworthiness and Transparency

Trust is essential in the midwife-client relationship. But for trauma survivors, trust is often broken. They may have been harmed by people they were supposed to trust, including family members or previous healthcare providers. They may be hypervigilant for signs that you are not trustworthy.

You cannot demand trust. You must earn it.

Trustworthiness means being honest, transparent, and accountable. It means doing what you say you are going to do.

In midwifery practice, building trustworthiness means:

- **Transparency in Decision-Making:** Explaining the rationale behind recommendations and policies. Being honest about the limits of your knowledge or the uncertainties of a situation. If you recommend an induction, explain why, what the risks and benefits are, and what the alternatives are.
- **Clear Communication:** Using clear, accessible language and avoiding jargon. Ensuring that the patient understands the information provided.
- **Informed Consent as an Ongoing Process:** Not just getting a signature on a form, but engaging in a continuous dialogue about risks, benefits, and alternatives. Consent can be revoked at any time.
- **Accountability:** Taking responsibility for mistakes and apologizing when necessary. If you mess up, own it. Don't make excuses.

3. Peer Support

Peer support is about connecting with people who have shared lived experiences. For trauma survivors, knowing that they are not alone and that others have survived similar experiences can be incredibly healing. Trauma is isolating. Peer support breaks that isolation.

In midwifery practice, facilitating peer support means:

- **Group Prenatal Care:** Offering group prenatal care models (like CenteringPregnancy), where people can connect with other expectant parents.
- **Support Groups:** Connecting clients with support groups for trauma survivors, birth trauma survivors, or new parents.
- **Lived Experience:** Hiring staff who have lived experience of trauma or perinatal mental health challenges (when appropriate and ethically managed).
- **Community Resources:** Valuing the wisdom and experience of community-based doulas and birth workers.

4. Collaboration and Mutuality

Traditional healthcare is often hierarchical. The provider holds the power and makes the decisions. This dynamic is inherently re-traumatizing for trauma survivors, who often experienced a deep loss of power and control during their trauma.

Collaboration and mutuality mean shifting the power dynamic. It means recognizing that the client is the expert on their own body and experience. It means partnering with the client to make decisions about their care.

In midwifery practice, fostering collaboration means:

- **Shared Decision-Making:** Presenting options and supporting the client in making the choices that are right for them, even if they differ from your recommendations. Stop telling people what they are "allowed" to do.
- **Respecting Autonomy:** Honoring the client's right to make decisions about their body and their birth.
- **Leveling the Playing Field:** Sitting at the same eye level as the client, wearing street clothes instead of scrubs (if appropriate for the setting), and asking them what they would like to be called.

- **Valuing the Client's Expertise:** Asking about their preferences, needs, and goals for their care. "What is most important to you today?" "What has helped you in the past?"

5. Agency, Voice, and Choice

Let's talk about power. Trauma is fundamentally about a loss of power. It involves a loss of control, autonomy, and agency. The goal of trauma-informed care is to restore agency to the survivor by prioritizing their voice and their choices.

We want to support the client in recognizing their own strengths and capabilities, and in taking control of their own health and healing.

Voice means ensuring that the client has the opportunity to express their needs, preferences, and concerns, and that their voice is heard and respected.

Choice means providing the client with options and alternatives, and respecting their right to make decisions about their own care, including the right to refuse care.

In maternity care, this is absolutely critical. Birthing people often feel like their bodies are not their own, that they have no say in what happens to them.

In practice, this looks like:

- **Offering Choices:** Providing choices whenever possible, even small ones. "Would you like the blood pressure cuff on your left or right arm?" "Would you prefer to sit up or lie down for this exam?" Small choices build a sense of control.
- **Validation:** Letting the client know that their feelings are valid and that they have a right to feel the way they do. "It makes sense that you are feeling scared, given what happened last time."
- **Strengths-Based Approach:** Focusing on the client's strengths and resilience, rather than just their deficits and pathology.

- **Supporting Self-Advocacy:** Helping the client develop the skills and confidence to advocate for themselves in the healthcare system.

This principle challenges the idea that the provider always knows best. It requires humility and a willingness to relinquish control.

6. Cultural, Historical, and Gender Issues

Trauma does not occur in a vacuum. It is shaped by the cultural, historical, and social context in which it occurs. A trauma-informed approach must acknowledge and address the impact of systemic oppression, discrimination, and historical trauma.

This principle requires us to move beyond cultural competence, which often focuses on superficial aspects of culture, to *cultural humility*. Cultural humility is a lifelong process of self-reflection and self-critique, where we acknowledge our own biases and assumptions, and commit to learning from our clients (Tervalon & Murray-García, 1998).

In practice, this looks like:

- **Recognizing Bias:** Acknowledging that we all have biases, and actively working to identify and address how our biases impact our practice.
- **Addressing Racism and Discrimination:** Recognizing the reality of racial trauma and the impact of racism on health outcomes. Providing anti-racist care that acknowledges and addresses the systemic inequities that marginalized communities face.
- **Gender-Affirming Care:** Providing care that is affirming and respectful of all gender identities. This means using correct names and pronouns, avoiding assumptions about gender roles and family structures, and understanding the unique needs of LGBTQIA+ birthing people.
- **Historical Context:** Understanding the historical context of trauma in specific communities, such as the history of medical abuse and exploitation of BIPOC communities.

31

- **Accessibility:** Ensuring that care is accessible to all people, regardless of their language, literacy level, disability status, or socioeconomic background.

If you ignore the impact of systemic oppression, you are not providing trauma-informed care. It's that simple.

The Four R's Realizing Recognizing Responding and Resisting Re-traumatization

In addition to the six principles, SAMHSA also describes the "Four R's" as a guide for implementing a trauma-informed approach (SAMHSA, 2014). These are the actions that organizations and individuals need to take.

1. Realizing

The first step is *realizing* the widespread impact of trauma and understanding the potential paths for recovery. This means educating yourself and your colleagues about the prevalence of trauma, the neurobiology of trauma, and the principles of TIC.

2. Recognizing

The second step is *recognizing* the signs and symptoms of trauma in clients, families, staff, and others involved with the system. As we discussed in Chapter 2, this means being attuned to the subtle cues of hyperarousal, dissociation, and avoidance.

It also means recognizing the signs of vicarious trauma and burnout in yourself and your colleagues.

3. Responding

The third step is *responding* by fully integrating knowledge about trauma into policies, procedures, and practices. This is where the rubber meets the road. It's not enough to just understand trauma; you have to change how you practice.

Responding means applying the principles of TIC in every interaction. It means:

- Using trauma-informed communication strategies.
- Implementing protocols for consent and choice.
- Creating a physically and psychologically safe environment.
- Providing appropriate referrals for trauma-specific treatment when needed.

4. Resisting Re-traumatization

The fourth step is actively *resisting re-traumatization*. This means identifying and eliminating practices that may inadvertently cause harm or trigger trauma responses.

The healthcare system is full of potentially re-traumatizing practices. Invasive procedures without consent, disrespectful communication, lack of privacy, and rigid adherence to policies—all of these can mirror the dynamics of past trauma and cause further injury.

Resisting re-traumatization requires a constant process of self-reflection and quality improvement. It means asking yourself and your colleagues: "Is this practice safe? Does it support autonomy? Is it collaborative?"

Challenges in Implementing TIC

Look, I'm not going to sugarcoat it. Implementing trauma-informed care is hard. It requires a significant commitment of time, energy, and emotional labor. You will likely encounter resistance.

Some common challenges include:

- **Time Constraints:** You might think, "I don't have time for this." But the reality is, you don't have time *not* to do this. Dealing with the fallout of re-traumatization takes much more time and energy in the long run.

- **Lack of Training and Resources:** Many healthcare professionals have not received adequate training in TIC.
- **Resistance to Change:** People are often resistant to changing the way they have always done things. You may hear comments like, "We don't have time for this touchy-feely stuff."
- **Systemic Barriers:** The healthcare system is often designed for efficiency and risk management, rather than individualized care.
- **Vicarious Trauma and Burnout:** Working with trauma survivors can be emotionally taxing.

Overcoming the Challenges

Despite these challenges, implementing TIC is not only possible; it is essential. It is the ethical obligation of every healthcare provider.

Here are a few strategies for overcoming the barriers:

- **Start Small:** You don't have to change everything overnight. Start with small changes in your own practice. For example, you can start by asking for permission before touching a patient.
- **Build a Coalition:** Find allies in your workplace who are also committed to TIC.
- **Provide Education and Training:** Share what you are learning with your colleagues.
- **Focus on the Benefits:** Emphasize the benefits of TIC for both patients and providers. TIC can improve patient outcomes, increase patient satisfaction, and reduce staff burnout.
- **Be Patient and Persistent:** Change takes time. Be patient with yourself and your colleagues.

The Bottom Line

The principles of trauma-informed care are not revolutionary. They are simply the principles of good healthcare. They are what we should be doing for everyone, regardless of their trauma history.

When we practice trauma-informed care, we are not just avoiding harm. We are creating opportunities for healing. The perinatal period is a time of deep vulnerability, but it is also a time of incredible potential for growth and transformation. When we provide care that is safe, supportive, and collaborative, we can help people reclaim their bodies, their voices, and their lives.

In the next part of this book, we will move from principles to practice. We will look at concrete strategies and skills for applying TIC in the clinical setting.

Key Takeaways

- Trauma-informed care (TIC) is a fundamental shift in approach, moving from "What's wrong with you?" to "What happened to you?"

- The six core principles of TIC are Safety; Trustworthiness and Transparency; Peer Support; Collaboration and Mutuality; Agency, Voice, and Choice; and Cultural, Historical, and Gender Issues.

- Safety is the foundation of TIC and includes both physical and psychological safety.

- Collaboration and supporting autonomy mean shifting the power dynamic and recognizing the client as the expert on their own body and experience.

- The Four R's (Realizing, Recognizing, Responding, and Resisting Re-traumatization) provide a guide for implementing TIC.

- Resisting re-traumatization means actively identifying and eliminating practices that may cause harm or trigger trauma responses.

- Implementing TIC is challenging but essential for providing ethical and effective care.

Chapter 4: Creating Safety in Clinical Encounters

We've established that safety is the foundation of trauma-informed care. If the nervous system doesn't feel safe, the thinking brain stays offline, the stress response is activated, and the risk of re-traumatization is high.

But what does "creating safety" actually look like? It's not just about preventing physical harm. It's about the subtle cues—the environment, your demeanor, your language—that communicate to the client's nervous system: "You are safe here. You are respected. You are in control."

This chapter is about the practical, concrete strategies you can use to create safety in every clinical encounter, whether it's a routine prenatal visit or the intensity of labor. This stuff isn't complicated. But it requires mindfulness and a willingness to change habits that are deeply ingrained in the culture of healthcare.

The Physical Environment

The physical environment plays a huge role in how safe a person feels. Trauma survivors are often hyper-attuned to their surroundings, constantly scanning for potential threats (even if they aren't consciously aware of it). A chaotic, stressful environment can trigger a trauma response before you even say a word.

Lighting

Bright, harsh lighting, especially fluorescent lighting, can be overstimulating and anxiety-provoking. It can make people feel exposed and vulnerable. Think about the difference between the lighting in a cozy living room and the lighting in an interrogation room. We want our clinical spaces to feel more like the former.

Action Steps:

- Use natural light whenever possible.

- Install dimmer switches on overhead lights.

- Use lamps with soft, warm bulbs instead of overhead lighting during appointments and labor.

- During labor, keep the room dimly lit to promote oxytocin release and create a sense of privacy.

Sound

Loud, sudden noises can be startling and triggering. The constant beep of monitors, the chatter of staff in the hallways, the squeak of wheels on the floor—all of these can contribute to a sense of chaos and unsafety.

Action Steps:

- Minimize unnecessary noise in the clinical environment. Close doors quietly.

- Speak in a calm, quiet voice.

- Offer earplugs or noise-canceling headphones to clients.

- If possible, adjust the volume on monitors and alarms so they are audible but not jarring.

- Be mindful of conversations happening outside the client's room. Don't talk about other patients or personal matters where you can be overheard.

Minimizing Intrusion

In the hospital setting, intrusions are constant. People coming and going, knocking on the door, entering without permission. This can be incredibly disruptive to the labor process and triggering for trauma survivors, who may feel trapped and unable to protect their space.

Action Steps:

- **Knock and Wait:** Knock before entering the room and wait for a response. Don't just barge in.
- **Introduce Yourself:** Introduce yourself and explain your role every time you enter the room. "Hi, I'm Sarah, I'm the nurse who will be taking care of you today."
- **Minimize Numbers:** Minimize the number of people in the room. Ask the client who they want present.
- **Cluster Care:** Cluster care activities (e.g., vital signs, medication administration) to minimize interruptions.
- **Privacy Signs:** Use signs on the door to indicate the client is resting or requests privacy.

Spatial Awareness

Trauma survivors often have a heightened sensitivity to personal space. Feeling crowded, trapped, or touched unexpectedly can trigger a fight or flight response.

Action Steps:

- **Clear Exit:** Arrange the room so the client has a clear path to the exit. Don't block the door.
- **Eye Level:** Sit at the same eye level as the client, rather than standing over them. This reduces the power differential.
- **Respectful Distance:** Maintain a respectful distance when talking to the client. Avoid looming or crowding.
- **Ask Permission:** Ask for permission before entering the client's personal space. "Is it okay if I sit next to you?"
- **Body Language:** Be mindful of your body language. Avoid crossed arms, tense posture, or sudden movements.

The Emotional Environment

The emotional environment is just as important as the physical environment. It is created by the attitudes, behaviors, and interactions of the staff. A warm, welcoming, and respectful emotional environment can help regulate the nervous system and build trust.

Demeanor

Your demeanor—your facial expressions, your tone of voice, your energy—communicates volumes to your clients. If you are rushed, stressed, or distracted, your client will pick up on it and feel unsafe. Remember co-regulation from Chapter 2? Your nervous system communicates with their nervous system.

Action Steps:

- **Ground Yourself:** Take a deep breath before entering the room and consciously ground yourself. Leave your stress outside the door.
- **Eye Contact:** Make eye contact (if culturally appropriate and comfortable for the client).
- **Warm Greeting:** Offer a warm smile and a genuine greeting.
- **Calm Presence:** Maintain a calm, regulated presence, even in stressful situations. If an emergency happens, you need to be the calmest person in the room.

Pacing

The pace of modern healthcare is often frantic. Rushed appointments, rapid-fire questions, quick procedures. This fast pace can be overwhelming and triggering for trauma survivors, who may need more time to process information and make decisions.

Action Steps:

- **Slow Down:** Seriously. Slow down. Speak slowly and clearly.
- **Allow Silence:** Allow silence and pauses in the conversation. Don't rush to fill every gap.
- **Time to Process:** Give the client time to think and respond to questions. Don't interrupt them.

- **Step-by-Step Explanation:** Explain what is happening step-by-step and check for understanding.
- **Acknowledge Rush:** If you are feeling rushed, acknowledge it and apologize. "I know this feels rushed. I want to make sure we have enough time to address your concerns."

Non-Verbal Communication

Non-verbal communication is powerful. It can either build safety or erode it.

Action Steps:

- **Open Posture:** Maintain an open, relaxed posture.
- **Active Listening:** Nod and use active listening cues to show you are engaged.
- **Mindful Expressions:** Be mindful of your facial expressions. Avoid expressions of judgment, frustration, or disbelief.
- **Intentional Touch:** Use touch intentionally and respectfully, always asking for permission first.

Language that Heals vs Language that Harms

The words we use matter. Language can be a tool for healing or a weapon for harm. Trauma-informed communication involves using language that is respectful, supportive of agency, and non-judgmental.

Avoiding Judgmental and Labeling Language

Labels like "non-compliant," "difficult," "attention-seeking," or "drug-seeking" are harmful and counterproductive. They blame the client for their behavior and ignore the underlying reasons for it. These labels are often rooted in bias and assumptions.

- **Instead of:** "She's being non-compliant with her diabetes management."
- **Try:** "She's facing challenges with managing her diabetes. Let's explore what's getting in the way."

Avoiding Coercive and Threatening Language

Coercion and threats are never acceptable in healthcare. They erode trust and can be deeply re-traumatizing. This includes subtle coercion, like using guilt or fear to persuade a client to agree to a procedure.

- **Instead of:** "If you don't do this test, your baby could be in danger." (Fear-based coercion)
- **Try:** "This test is recommended because it gives us information about your baby's well-being. Let's talk about the risks and benefits and what feels right for you."

Using Language that Supports Agency

Use language that emphasizes choice, collaboration, and respect for autonomy.

- **Instead of:** "I need you to lie down so I can examine you."
- **Try:** "For this exam, the best position is lying down. Are you comfortable doing that now?"

Using Invitations and Permissions

Use language that invites the client to participate in their care and asks for permission before acting.

- **Instead of:** "I'm going to check your blood pressure now."
- **Try:** "Is it okay if I check your blood pressure now?"

Using Clear and Accessible Language

Avoid medical jargon and use clear, simple language.

- **Instead of:** "We need to augment your labor due to failure to progress."
- **Try:** "Your labor seems to have slowed down. We can talk about ways to help it pick up again, like using medication to make your contractions stronger."

Sample Scripts for Trauma-Informed Communication

Here are some examples of trauma-informed language in practice:

Introducing yourself:
"Hi, my name is [Name], and I'm one of the midwives here. I'll be caring for you today. How would you like me to address you?"

Setting the agenda:
"We have about 20 minutes together today. I'd like to check on how you and the baby are doing, and I also want to make sure we have time to answer your questions and talk about what's important to you. How does that sound?"

Asking sensitive questions:
"Sometimes people have experiences in their past that make coming to the doctor or receiving medical care difficult. Is there anything you want me to know so I can provide you with the best possible care?"

Responding to distress:
"I can see that this is difficult for you. It's okay to feel overwhelmed. We can take a break if you need to. I'm here with you."

Building Trust and Rapport Quickly and Ethically

In a busy clinical setting, you often don't have a lot of time to build trust and rapport. But you can use the time you have intentionally to create a connection and establish a foundation of safety.

Start with Connection

Before diving into the clinical tasks, take a moment to connect with the client as a human being.

Action Steps:

- Acknowledge the client's presence and welcome them warmly.

- Ask a non-medical question to open the conversation. "How are you doing today, really?"
- Notice something positive about the client and comment on it genuinely (if appropriate and authentic).

Be Present and Attuned

Put down the chart. Turn away from the computer. Give the client your full attention. This is harder than it sounds in the age of electronic health records, but it is crucial.

Action Steps:

- **Active Listening:** Listen actively and reflectively. "What I hear you saying is..."
- **Validation:** Validate the client's feelings and experiences. "That sounds incredibly difficult."
- **Curiosity:** Be curious about the client's perspective. "Tell me more about that."

Be Transparent and Honest

Transparency builds trust. Be clear about what you are doing and why.

Action Steps:

- **Explain Purpose:** Explain the purpose of the appointment or procedure.
- **Narrate Actions:** Narrate your actions as you go. "I'm going to put this cuff on your arm. It will feel tight for a moment."
- **Honesty:** Be honest about the limitations of your knowledge or the uncertainties of the situation.

Offer Choices

Offering choices helps the client feel a sense of agency and control.

Action Steps:

- **Provide Options:** Provide options whenever possible, even small ones.
- **Respect Decisions:** Respect the client's decisions, even if you disagree with them.
- **Shared Decision-Making:** Use shared decision-making tools to facilitate collaboration.

Ethical Considerations

Building trust and rapport requires maintaining clear professional boundaries. Trauma survivors may have difficulty with boundaries due to their past experiences.

Action Steps:

- **Clear Roles:** Be clear about your role and the limits of your relationship.
- **Avoid Oversharing:** Avoid oversharing personal information.
- **Mindful of Transference:** Be mindful of transference and countertransference (the feelings that arise in the provider-client relationship based on past experiences).
- **Confidentiality:** Maintain confidentiality and explain the limits of confidentiality.

Case Example The Prenatal Appointment

Let's look at how these strategies come together in a prenatal appointment.

Jasmine is a 30-year-old pregnant with her first child. She has a history of childhood medical trauma. She arrives at the clinic looking tense and anxious.

The midwife, Alex, takes a deep breath before greeting her.

Alex: "Hi Jasmine, I'm Alex, one of the midwives. It's good to see you today. Please come in and sit wherever you feel most comfortable." (Warm greeting, spatial awareness)

Alex sits at the same eye level as Jasmine and maintains an open posture.

Alex: "We have about 15 minutes together today. I'd like to check how you're doing, listen to the baby's heartbeat, and measure your belly. But first, how are you feeling?" (Pacing, setting the agenda, connection)

Jasmine shares that she is feeling anxious about the appointment.

Alex: "Thank you for sharing that with me. It makes sense that you would feel anxious, given your past experiences. I want you to know that you are in control here. We can go at your pace, and we can stop at any time if you need to." (Validation, supporting agency)

When it's time for the physical exam, Alex explains what she is going to do step-by-step and asks for permission before touching Jasmine.

Alex: "Is it okay if I measure your belly now? It involves me pressing gently on your abdomen with the tape measure." (Transparency, consent)

During the exam, Alex notices Jasmine holding her breath.

Alex: "Jasmine, I notice you're holding your breath. It's okay to breathe. If you like, we can take a deep breath together." (Attunement, co-regulation)

At the end of the appointment, Alex summarizes the plan and checks for understanding.

Alex: "So, we talked about [X, Y, Z]. How does that sound to you? What questions do you have?" (Collaboration, clarity)

By intentionally creating safety and building trust, Alex helps Jasmine stay within her window of tolerance and have a positive experience of care.

The Ongoing Work of Safety

Creating safety is not a one-time event. It is an ongoing process that requires constant attention and effort. You will make mistakes. You will inadvertently trigger clients. The key is to recognize when this happens, take responsibility for it, and repair the rupture in the relationship.

In the next chapter, we will look at how to assess for trauma history and symptoms in a way that is safe, ethical, and supportive of agency.

Key Takeaways

- Creating safety is the foundation of trauma-informed care. It involves small, intentional actions that communicate safety and respect.

- The physical environment should be calm, predictable, and minimize triggers (e.g., soft lighting, minimal noise, minimizing intrusions).

- The emotional environment should be warm, welcoming, and respectful (e.g., calm demeanor, slow pacing, mindful non-verbal communication).

- Language should be respectful, supportive of agency, and non-judgmental. Avoid coercive or labeling language. Use invitations and permissions.

- Building trust and rapport requires presence, attunement, transparency, and offering choices, while maintaining ethical boundaries.

- Creating safety is an ongoing process that requires mindfulness, intentionality, and a willingness to change habits.

Chapter 5: Trauma Assessment Tools and Screening

Now we get to a tricky area: screening and assessment for trauma. On the one hand, we know that trauma is common and that it significantly impacts perinatal health. Identifying trauma history and symptoms can help us tailor our care and provide appropriate support and referrals.

On the other hand, asking about trauma can be incredibly sensitive. If done poorly, it can be triggering, re-traumatizing, and damaging to the provider-client relationship.

The goal of trauma screening and assessment in the midwifery setting is not to diagnose PTSD or to force clients to disclose their trauma history. The goal is to identify those who may be at risk for trauma-related difficulties and to open the door for supportive conversations and interventions.

This chapter will explore the ethics of screening, the different approaches to assessment, recommended tools, and practical strategies for asking sensitive questions in a trauma-informed way.

The Ethics of Screening Universal Precautions vs Direct Inquiry

There are two main approaches to addressing trauma in healthcare settings: universal precautions and direct inquiry.

Universal Precautions

Universal precautions means assuming that everyone may have a history of trauma and providing trauma-informed care to all clients, regardless of whether they disclose a trauma history. This approach is based on the principles of TIC that we discussed in Chapter 3: safety, trustworthiness, collaboration, agency, and choice.

The advantage of universal precautions is that it minimizes the risk of re-traumatization. Clients do not have to disclose their trauma history to receive respectful and supportive care. It also recognizes that many people may not identify their experiences as traumatic, or may not feel safe disclosing them.

Universal precautions are the foundation of trauma-informed midwifery care. Even if you choose to implement direct screening, you must always practice universal precautions.

Direct Inquiry (Screening)

Direct inquiry involves asking clients directly about their trauma history and symptoms using standardized screening tools or clinical interviews.

The advantage of direct inquiry is that it can help identify specific needs and risks that might otherwise be missed. It can also validate the client's experiences and normalize the conversation about trauma.

However, direct inquiry also carries risks. It can be triggering for clients, especially if they are not prepared for the questions or if the provider is not trained to respond appropriately. It can also create a sense of pressure to disclose, which can undermine agency.

The Ethical Imperative Do No Harm

If you choose to implement direct screening for trauma, you must do so ethically and responsibly. This means ensuring that the following conditions are met:

1. **Safety and Privacy:** Screening must be conducted in a safe, private, and confidential setting. Clients must be informed about how their information will be used and protected.
2. **Informed Consent:** Clients must be informed about the purpose of the screening and have the right to decline without consequence.
3. **Provider Training:** Providers must be trained in trauma-informed communication, how to respond to disclosures of trauma, and how to provide appropriate referrals.

4. **Resources and Referrals:** Organizations must have resources in place to support clients who screen positive for trauma. This includes access to trauma-specific treatment and support services.

If you cannot ensure these conditions are met, you should not be screening for trauma. Asking about trauma without the ability to respond appropriately is unethical and harmful.

Recommended Assessment Tools

There are many tools available for screening and assessing trauma. The choice of tool depends on the setting, the population, and the goals of the assessment.

Adverse Childhood Experiences (ACEs)

The ACEs questionnaire is a 10-item tool that screens for experiences of abuse, neglect, and household dysfunction during childhood (Felitti et al., 1998).

- **Pros:** It is quick and easy to administer. It provides a measure of cumulative childhood adversity, which is linked to long-term health outcomes.
- **Cons:** It does not assess for trauma experienced in adulthood. It does not assess for the impact of the experiences (the effects). Some clients may find the questions intrusive.

PTSD Checklist for DSM-5 (PCL-5)

The PCL-5 is a 20-item self-report measure that assesses the symptoms of PTSD based on the DSM-5 criteria (Weathers et al., 2013).

- **Pros:** It is a validated and reliable measure of PTSD symptoms. It can be used to screen for PTSD and monitor symptoms over time.
- **Cons:** It is longer than some other screening tools. It focuses on symptoms, not the history of trauma.

Perinatal PTSD Questionnaire (PPQ)

The PPQ is a 14-item self-report measure specifically designed to screen for postpartum PTSD (Callahan et al., 2006).

- **Pros:** It is specifically tailored to the perinatal population. It focuses on symptoms related to the birth experience.
- **Cons:** It is not as widely validated as the PCL-5.

Adaptations and Considerations

When using these tools, it is important to consider the specific needs of the perinatal population. For example, when using the PCL-5 during pregnancy, you might want to adapt the instructions to focus on current symptoms or symptoms related to past trauma that are impacting the pregnancy.

It is also important to recognize that these tools are just one piece of the puzzle. They should be used in conjunction with clinical judgment and a comprehensive assessment.

The Art of Inquiry How to Ask Sensitive Questions Without Re-traumatizing

How you ask about trauma is just as important as what you ask. The goal is to invite the client to share their experiences in a way that feels safe, respectful, and supportive of agency.

Preparing the Client

Before asking sensitive questions, it is important to prepare the client and obtain their consent.

- **Normalize the Inquiry:** Explain that you ask these questions to everyone because you know that many people have experienced difficult things in their lives.

- *Example:* "Because experiences in our past can affect our health and well-being, we ask all of our clients about things like violence, abuse, and trauma."
- **Explain the Purpose:** Explain why you are asking these questions and how the information will be used.
  - *Example:* "We ask these questions so we can better understand your needs and provide you with the best possible care."
- **Ensure Confidentiality:** Reassure the client that their information will be kept confidential, and explain the limits of confidentiality (e.g., mandatory reporting requirements).
  - *Example:* "Everything you share with me is confidential, unless you tell me that you are planning to hurt yourself or someone else, or if there is a concern about the safety of a child."
- **Offer Choice and Control:** Emphasize that the client has the right to decline to answer any questions and that they can stop the conversation at any time.
  - *Example:* "You don't have to answer any questions you don't want to. And if you want to stop talking about this at any time, just let me know."

Asking the Questions

When asking the questions, use a calm, compassionate, and non-judgmental tone of voice.

- **Use Clear and Direct Language:** Avoid euphemisms or jargon.
- **Be Specific:** Ask about specific behaviors rather than using labels like "abuse" or "trauma."
- **Pace the Conversation:** Go slowly and allow the client time to process the questions and their responses.
- **Be Attuned to the Client's Response:** Pay attention to the client's body language, tone of voice, and emotional reactions. If the client becomes distressed, stop the conversation and offer support.

Examples of Trauma-Informed Questions

Here are some examples of questions you can use to inquire about trauma in a trauma-informed way:

- **General Inquiry:**
    - "Is there anything in your past that makes receiving medical care difficult or uncomfortable for you?"
    - "Are there any procedures or exams that you are particularly worried about?"
- **Childhood Adversity (ACEs):**
    - "While you were growing up, did you ever feel unsafe in your home?"
    - "Did anyone in your household ever hit, beat, kick, or physically hurt you in any way?"
- **Intimate Partner Violence (IPV):**
    - "Do you feel safe in your current relationship?"
    - "Has your partner ever threatened you, hurt you, or forced you to do something you didn't want to do?"
- **Birth Trauma:**
    - "How would you describe your previous birth experience?"
    - "Were there any moments during your labor or birth when you felt scared, helpless, or out of control?"

Responding to Disclosures Validation Support and Appropriate Referrals

When a client discloses a history of trauma, how you respond is critical. Your response can either support healing or cause further harm.

The Four C's of Responding to Disclosure

1. **Calm:** Maintain a calm, regulated presence. Avoid reacting with shock, horror, or pity.

2. **Compassion:** Express empathy and compassion for the client's experiences.
3. **Curiosity:** Be curious about the client's needs and how you can support them.
4. **Connection:** Reassure the client that they are not alone and that help is available.

Validation

Validation is the most important part of responding to a disclosure. It means acknowledging the client's experiences and feelings without judgment.

- **Believe the Client:** Start by believing the client's story. Avoid questioning or minimizing their experiences.
- **Acknowledge the Difficulty of Disclosure:** Thank the client for trusting you enough to share their story.
- **Normalize the Response:** Reassure the client that their feelings and reactions are normal and understandable given what they have been through.

Examples of Validating Statements:

- "Thank you for sharing that with me. I know it can be difficult to talk about."

- "I'm so sorry that happened to you. It sounds incredibly painful."

- "It makes sense that you would feel scared/angry/anxious given what you've been through."

- "You are not alone. Many people have had similar experiences."

- "It was not your fault."

Support

After validating the client's experiences, offer support and reassurance.

- **Assess Immediate Safety:** If the client is in immediate danger (e.g., experiencing active IPV or suicidal ideation), follow your organization's protocols for safety planning and intervention.
- **Address Immediate Needs:** Ask the client what they need in the moment to feel safe and supported.
  - *Example:* "What can I do right now to help you feel safe?"
- **Collaborate on a Plan of Care:** Work with the client to develop a plan of care that addresses their needs and preferences.
  - *Example:* "Given what you've shared with me, let's talk about how we can make your prenatal care and birth experience feel as safe and comfortable as possible."

Appropriate Referrals

Midwives are not expected to be trauma therapists. However, we have a responsibility to connect clients with appropriate resources and referrals for trauma-specific treatment and support.

- **Know Your Resources:** Be familiar with the resources available in your community, such as therapists specializing in trauma and perinatal mental health, support groups, domestic violence shelters, and sexual assault crisis centers.
- **Offer Options:** Provide the client with information about the different types of resources available and let them choose what feels right for them.
- **Facilitate the Referral Process:** Offer to help the client make the initial contact with the resource, if they wish.
- **Follow Up:** Check in with the client at subsequent appointments about their experience with the referral and offer ongoing support.

Case Example Responding to a Disclosure

Let's look at an example of how to respond to a disclosure of trauma in a trauma-informed way.

During a prenatal appointment, you ask your client, Maya, if she has any concerns about the upcoming birth. Maya hesitates and then says, "I don't know if I can do this. I was sexually assaulted in college, and I'm terrified of the pain and the exams."

Trauma-Informed Response:

Midwife: "Maya, thank you so much for sharing that with me. I know that takes a lot of courage. I'm so sorry that happened to you. (Validation) It makes perfect sense that you would be feeling terrified about the birth, given your past experience. (Normalization) I want you to know that we can work together to make this experience feel as safe and supportive as possible for you. (Support)

"What would be helpful for us to talk about right now? We can talk about ways to cope with the pain, strategies for making exams feel safer, or anything else that is on your mind." (Collaboration)

If Maya expresses interest in therapy, the midwife can provide a referral.

Midwife: "Many survivors find it helpful to talk to a therapist who specializes in trauma and perinatal mental health. I have a list of resources here if you are interested. We can look at it together, or you can take it home and look at it later." (Referral, Choice)

Wrapping Up

Trauma screening and assessment are complex processes that require sensitivity, skill, and ethical awareness. By prioritizing universal precautions, using validated tools thoughtfully, asking sensitive questions in a trauma-informed way, and responding to disclosures with compassion and competence, we can identify clients who need extra support and create opportunities for healing and resilience.

In the next chapter, we will focus on the critical issues of consent, choice, and body autonomy in the context of trauma-informed midwifery care.

Key Takeaways

- Universal precautions (providing trauma-informed care to everyone) are the foundation of trauma-informed midwifery care.

- Direct inquiry (screening) can be helpful for identifying specific needs, but it must be done ethically and responsibly (safety, consent, training, resources).

- Recommended assessment tools include the ACEs questionnaire, the PCL-5, and the PPQ.

- When asking sensitive questions, prepare the client, normalize the inquiry, ensure confidentiality, and offer choice and control.

- Use clear, direct, and non-judgmental language.

- When responding to disclosures, prioritize validation, support, and appropriate referrals.

- The Four C's of responding to disclosure are Calm, Compassion, Curiosity, and Connection.

Chapter 6: Protocols for Consent, Choice, and Body Autonomy

If safety is the foundation of trauma-informed care, then consent, choice, and body autonomy are the pillars. Trauma is fundamentally about a violation of the self—a loss of control over one's body and experience. Therefore, restoring control, choice, and autonomy is central to the healing process.

In maternity care, these issues are particularly salient. Pregnancy and birth involve deep physical and emotional vulnerability. The potential for violation and re-traumatization is high. Standard practices often prioritize the provider's convenience or the institution's policies over the birthing person's autonomy.

This chapter will explore the concept of informed consent as an ongoing process, provide specific protocols for intimate examinations, discuss models for supporting agency and shared decision-making, and address the challenges of respecting body autonomy during necessary interventions.

This is not just about legal requirements. It's about ethical practice. It's about recognizing the inherent dignity and worth of every person we care for.

Informed Consent as an Ongoing Process (Not a One-Time Form)

Informed consent is a legal and ethical requirement in healthcare. But in practice, it often becomes a bureaucratic formality—a signature on a form that the client barely reads or understands.

A trauma-informed approach to informed consent recognizes that it is not a one-time event, but an ongoing process of communication, collaboration, and shared decision-making.

The Elements of True Informed Consent

True informed consent involves several key elements:

1. **Disclosure:** The provider must disclose all relevant information about the proposed procedure or treatment, including the benefits, risks, alternatives, and the consequences of doing nothing.
2. **Comprehension:** The client must understand the information provided. This means using clear, accessible language and checking for understanding.
3. **Capacity:** The client must have the capacity to make a decision. This means they must be able to understand the information and weigh the options. (Note: Laboring people generally have the capacity to make decisions, even if they are in pain or distressed.)
4. **Voluntariness:** The client must make the decision voluntarily, without coercion, manipulation, or undue influence.

Trauma-Informed Consent in Practice

A trauma-informed approach to consent emphasizes voluntariness and collaboration. It recognizes that trauma survivors may have difficulty saying no or expressing their preferences, especially in situations where there is a power differential (remember the fawn response from Chapter 2).

Here are some strategies for practicing trauma-informed consent:

- **Present Options, Not Directives:** Instead of telling the client what to do, present the options and invite them to participate in the decision-making process.
  - *Example:* "There are several options for managing your pain. Let's talk about them and see what feels right for you."
- **Use the BRAIN Acronym:** The BRAIN acronym is a useful tool for structuring informed consent discussions:

- o Benefits: What are the benefits of this procedure/treatment?
  - o Risks: What are the risks?
  - o Alternatives: What are the alternatives?
  - o Intuition: What does your intuition tell you?
  - o Nothing: What if we do nothing, or wait?
- **Check for Understanding:** Ask the client to summarize the information in their own words to ensure comprehension.
- **Allow Time for Reflection:** Give the client time to process the information and make a decision. Avoid rushing the conversation.
- **Respect the Right to Refuse:** Acknowledge and respect the client's right to refuse any procedure or treatment, even if you disagree with their decision.
- **Revisit Consent Frequently:** Consent is ongoing. The client has the right to change their mind at any time. Check in frequently to ensure the client is still comfortable with the plan of care.

Addressing Coercion

Coercion is the antithesis of informed consent. It involves using pressure, threats, or manipulation to force a client to comply with a recommendation. Coercion is common in maternity care, often disguised as concern for the baby's well-being.

Examples of coercive language:

- "If you don't do this, your baby might die."
- "You don't want to harm your baby, do you?"
- "We don't allow that here."
- "You just need to relax and let us do our job."

Coercion is unethical and harmful. It erodes trust and can be deeply re-traumatizing. We must actively identify and eliminate coercive practices in our care.

Protocols for Intimate Examinations

Intimate examinations, such as cervical checks, vaginal ultrasounds, and perineal repairs, are inherently invasive and vulnerable. For trauma survivors, particularly those with a history of sexual abuse, these procedures can be terrifying and triggering.

A trauma-informed approach to intimate examinations prioritizes the client's safety, comfort, and control.

Before the Exam

- **Explain the Purpose:** Clearly explain the purpose of the exam and why it is recommended.
- **Discuss Alternatives:** Discuss any alternatives to the exam, if applicable (e.g., other ways to assess labor progress instead of a cervical check).
- **Obtain Explicit Consent:** Ask for explicit verbal consent before starting the exam.
  - *Example:* "I'd like to offer a cervical check now to see how your labor is progressing. It involves me inserting two fingers into your vagina to feel your cervix. Are you okay with that?"
- **Offer Control:** Offer the client choices and control over the exam process.
  - *Example:* "Would you like to insert the speculum yourself?" "Would you prefer to be sitting up or lying down?"

During the Exam

- **Ensure Privacy:** Ensure the room is private and minimize the number of people present.
- **Use Trauma-Informed Techniques:**
  - Use adequate lubrication.
  - Warm the instruments (e.g., the speculum or ultrasound probe).

- Use the smallest size instrument appropriate for the exam.

- Go slowly and gently.

- **Narrate Your Actions:** Explain what you are doing step-by-step before you do it.
  - *Example:* "You're going to feel my hand on your leg now." "Now you will feel some pressure."
- **Check In Frequently:** Check in with the client throughout the exam to ensure they are comfortable and consent is ongoing.
  - *Example:* "How are you doing?" "Are you okay to continue?"
- **Establish a Stop Signal:** Establish a clear stop signal (e.g., a word or gesture) that the client can use if they want to stop the exam at any time.
  - *Example:* "If you want me to stop for any reason, just say 'stop,' and I will immediately remove my hands."
- **Respond to Distress:** If the client becomes distressed or triggered during the exam, stop immediately and offer support.

After the Exam

- **Provide Privacy to Get Dressed:** Leave the room or provide a private space for the client to get dressed.
- **Debrief the Experience:** Check in with the client about their experience of the exam.
  - *Example:* "How was that for you?"
- **Document the Process:** Document the consent process, the techniques used, and the client's response to the exam.

Case Example The Cervical Check

Let's look at an example of a trauma-informed cervical check.

Layla is in labor. She has a history of sexual abuse and has expressed anxiety about cervical checks.

Midwife: "Layla, your contractions are getting stronger and closer together. I'd like to offer a cervical check to see how your labor is progressing. This can help us make decisions about the next steps. How do you feel about that?" (Explaining purpose, offering choice)

Layla hesitates.

Layla: "I don't know. I hate them. They hurt so much."

Midwife: "I understand. They can be very uncomfortable. We can talk about ways to make it feel safer and more comfortable for you. For example, we can use a lot of lubricant, go very slowly, and you can choose the position that feels best for you. We can also establish a stop signal. If you say 'stop,' I will immediately stop." (Validation, offering control)

Layla agrees to try.

Midwife: "Okay. Before we start, let's take a deep breath together. I'm going to put some warm lubricant on my fingers. Now you're going to feel my hand on your thigh." (Pacing, narration)

During the exam, the midwife goes slowly and checks in frequently.

Midwife: "How are you doing? Are you okay to continue?"

If Layla says "stop," the midwife immediately removes her hands and offers support.

Midwife: "Okay, I'm stopping now. You did great. Let's take another deep breath. What do you need right now?"

Agency and Shared Decision-Making Models

Supporting agency and shared decision-making are core principles of trauma-informed care. They involve shifting the power dynamic from the provider as the expert to the client as the expert on their own body and experience.

Supporting Agency

Agency means supporting the client in recognizing their own strengths and capacities, and in taking control of their own health and healing.

- **Strengths-Based Approach:** Focus on the client's strengths and resilience, rather than their deficits.
- **Education and Information:** Provide the client with the information and resources they need to make informed decisions.
- **Skill Building:** Support the client in developing skills for self-advocacy, coping, and emotional regulation.
- **Belief in Recovery:** Communicate a belief in the client's ability to heal and thrive.

Shared Decision-Making (SDM)

Shared decision-making is a collaborative process where the provider and the client work together to make decisions about the plan of care. It involves integrating the provider's clinical expertise with the client's values, preferences, and goals.

The Three-Talk Model of SDM

The Three-Talk Model is a practical framework for implementing SDM in clinical practice (Elwyn et al., 2012):

1. **Team Talk:** Establish a collaborative relationship with the client. Emphasize that you are a team and that you will make decisions together.
2. **Option Talk:** Present the options, including the benefits, risks, and alternatives of each option. Use clear, balanced language and check for understanding.
3. **Decision Talk:** Support the client in exploring their preferences and values, and in making a decision that is right for them.

Example of the Three-Talk Model in Practice:

- **Team Talk:** "We need to make a decision about how to manage your blood pressure. I want us to work together as a team to figure out the best plan for you."
- **Option Talk:** "There are several options available, including medication, lifestyle changes, or a combination of both. Let's talk about the pros and cons of each option."
- **Decision Talk:** "Now that we've talked about the options, what are your thoughts? What is most important to you? How can I support you in making this decision?"

Respecting Body Autonomy Practices During Necessary Interventions

There are times when medical interventions are necessary to ensure the safety and well-being of the birthing person or the baby. These situations can be challenging because they often involve a loss of control and autonomy.

A trauma-informed approach to necessary interventions prioritizes minimizing harm, maximizing choice, and maintaining connection and communication throughout the process.

Minimizing Harm

- **Least Invasive Option:** Use the least invasive option that is clinically appropriate.
- **Pain Management:** Ensure adequate pain management during procedures.
- **Trauma-Informed Techniques:** Use trauma-informed techniques during procedures (e.g., gentle touch, clear communication).

Maximizing Choice

Even when interventions are necessary, there are often still choices available.

- **Timing:** Offer choices about the timing of the intervention, if possible.
- **Setting:** Offer choices about the environment (e.g., lighting, sound).
- **Support Persons:** Ensure the client has access to their support persons.
- **Small Choices:** Offer small choices throughout the process (e.g., which arm for the IV, what music to play).

Maintaining Connection and Communication

During emergencies or stressful procedures, communication often breaks down. Providers become focused on the clinical tasks and forget the human being in front of them. This can be terrifying and traumatizing for the client.

- **Continuous Communication:** Maintain continuous communication with the client throughout the procedure. Explain what is happening and why.
- **Emotional Support:** Offer emotional support and reassurance.
- **Eye Contact:** Maintain eye contact with the client, if possible.
- **Designated Support Person:** Assign a designated support person (e.g., a nurse or midwife) to stay with the client and provide continuous support and communication.

Case Example The Emergency C-Section

An emergency C-section is a high-stress situation where autonomy is often compromised. Here's how to apply trauma-informed principles in this scenario:

- **Clear Communication:** Explain the need for the C-section clearly and calmly. "The baby's heart rate is low, and we need to deliver the baby quickly to ensure their safety. We are going to do a C-section now."
- **Rapid Consent:** Obtain consent quickly but without coercion. "Do you consent to the C-section?"

- **Continuous Support:** Assign a nurse or midwife to stay with the birthing person and provide continuous support and communication.
- **Narrate the Process:** Explain what is happening step-by-step. "We are moving you to the operating room now." "You will feel some pressure during the surgery."
- **Maximize Connection:** Maintain eye contact and offer reassurance. "You are doing great. We are taking good care of you and your baby."
- **Facilitate Bonding:** Facilitate immediate skin-to-skin contact after the birth, if possible.
- **Debrief the Experience:** After the surgery, debrief the experience with the client and their family. Answer questions and validate their feelings.

Conclusion

Respecting consent, choice, and body autonomy is at the heart of trauma-informed midwifery care. It requires a fundamental shift in how we view our role as providers—from directors of care to partners in care.

By practicing informed consent as an ongoing process, implementing trauma-informed protocols for intimate examinations, fostering agency and shared decision-making, and respecting body autonomy even during necessary interventions, we can create a maternity care system that honors the dignity and worth of every birthing person.

In the next chapter, we will explore the important issues of documentation and communication in trauma-informed care.

Key Takeaways

- Informed consent is an ongoing process of communication and collaboration, not a one-time form.
- True informed consent requires disclosure, comprehension, capacity, and voluntariness.

- Coercion is unethical and harmful. We must actively identify and eliminate coercive practices.

- Protocols for intimate examinations should prioritize the client's safety, comfort, and control (e.g., explicit consent, narration of actions, stop signal).

- Supporting agency and shared decision-making involve shifting the power dynamic and recognizing the client as the expert on their own body and experience.

- The Three-Talk Model (Team Talk, Option Talk, Decision Talk) is a practical framework for implementing shared decision-making.

- During necessary interventions, prioritize minimizing harm, maximizing choice, and maintaining connection and communication.

Chapter 7: Documentation Considerations and Communication

Documentation is a critical aspect of healthcare. It serves as a record of the care provided, a communication tool between providers, and a legal document. However, documentation practices in healthcare often reflect the biases and assumptions of the providers and the system. They can perpetuate stigma, reinforce harmful stereotypes, and contribute to re-traumatization.

Trauma-informed documentation is about using language that is respectful, objective, strengths-based, and person-centered. It's about documenting the client's experience in a way that honors their dignity and promotes their well-being.

This chapter will explore the principles of trauma-informed documentation, provide strategies for avoiding judgmental and labeling language, discuss confidentiality protocols, and address the challenges of communicating trauma history sensitively in handovers and referrals.

Objective and Strengths-Based Documentation Practices

The traditional medical model of documentation often focuses on pathology and deficits. It emphasizes what is wrong with the client and what they are failing to do.

A trauma-informed approach to documentation shifts the focus to objectivity and strengths.

Objectivity

Objective documentation means recording the facts of the situation without interpretation or judgment. It means describing what you observed, heard, or measured, rather than your opinions or assumptions about the client's behavior.

- **Instead of:** "Client was angry and hostile during the appointment."
- **Try:** "Client was observed yelling, clenching fists, and stating, 'I am angry about the way I am being treated.'"
- **Instead of:** "Client refused the cervical exam."
- **Try:** "Client declined the cervical exam, stating, 'I do not want to do that right now.'"

Strengths-Based Approach

Strengths-based documentation means recognizing and highlighting the client's strengths, resilience, and coping strategies. It means focusing on what the client is doing well, rather than just their challenges.

- **Instead of:** "Client has a history of substance abuse and poor coping skills."
- **Try:** "Client reports a history of substance use disorder and is actively engaged in recovery. Client demonstrates resilience and commitment to their health and well-being."
- **Instead of:** "Client is struggling to bond with the baby."
- **Try:** "Client is adjusting to the demands of new parenthood and is actively seeking support to strengthen their connection with the baby. Client demonstrates attentiveness to the baby's cues."

Person-Centered Language

Person-centered language means putting the person first, rather than their diagnosis or condition. It means using language that is respectful and inclusive.

- **Instead of:** "Diabetic patient."
- **Try:** "Person with diabetes."
- **Instead of:** "Addict."
- **Try:** "Person with a substance use disorder."

Trauma-Informed Language

When documenting trauma history or symptoms, use language that is sensitive and non-stigmatizing.

- **Instead of:** "Victim of abuse."
- **Try:** "Survivor of abuse" or "Person who has experienced abuse." (Note: Some people prefer the term "survivor," while others prefer "person who has experienced." Ask the client what language they prefer, if possible.)
- **Instead of:** "Client claims to have been sexually assaulted."
- **Try:** "Client reports a history of sexual assault." (Using the word "claims" implies doubt. We should believe the client's report.)

Avoiding Labeling and Judgmental Language

Judgmental and labeling language is common in healthcare documentation. It reflects the provider's biases and assumptions and can have serious consequences for the client's care.

Common Labels to Avoid

- Non-compliant
- Difficult
- Resistant
- Manipulative
- Attention-seeking
- Drug-seeking
- Frequent flyer
- Poor historian

These labels are subjective, stigmatizing, and unhelpful. They blame the client for their behavior and ignore the underlying reasons for it.

Focus on Behavior, Not Personality

Instead of using labels to describe the client's personality, focus on describing their behavior objectively.

- **Instead of:** "Client is manipulative."
- **Try:** "Client requested pain medication before the scheduled time, stating, 'I need something stronger.'"

Consider the Context

When documenting behavior, consider the context in which it occurred. What might be driving the behavior? Is it a response to stress, fear, or trauma?

- **Example:** "Client became agitated during the cervical exam, stating, 'Stop, I can't do this.' Client appeared fearful and tense. Provider stopped the exam and offered support. Client reported a history of sexual abuse."

The Impact of Judgmental Language

Judgmental language in documentation can have serious consequences:

- **Stigma:** It can create stigma and prejudice against the client, affecting how they are treated by other providers.
- **Bias:** It can reinforce biases and stereotypes, leading to disparities in care.
- **Erosion of Trust:** It can damage the provider-client relationship and erode trust in the healthcare system.
- **Re-traumatization:** It can be re-traumatizing for the client to read judgmental language about themselves in their medical record (especially with open access to notes).

A Note on "Non-Compliant" and "Refused"

The terms "non-compliant" and "refused" are particularly problematic.

"Non-compliant" implies that the client is willfully disobeying the provider's orders. It ignores the fact that the client has the right to make decisions about their own care, and that there may be valid reasons for their choices.

- **Instead of:** "Non-compliant with medication."
- **Try:** "Declined medication due to concerns about side effects."

"Refused" can sound harsh and adversarial. It implies a confrontation rather than a choice.

- **Instead of:** "Refused induction of labor."
- **Try:** "Declined induction of labor, preferring to wait for spontaneous labor."

Using the word "declined" instead of "refused" is a simple shift that honors the client's autonomy and respects their decision-making process.

Confidentiality Protocols

Confidentiality is a cornerstone of ethical healthcare practice. It is essential for building trust and creating a safe space for clients to disclose sensitive information.

Informed Consent for Information Sharing

Clients must be informed about how their information will be used and shared, and they must provide informed consent for any sharing of information outside the healthcare team.

Action Steps:

- Explain your organization's confidentiality policies clearly and concisely.
- Obtain written consent for sharing information with external providers or agencies.

- Reassure the client that their information will be protected.

Limits of Confidentiality

There are limits to confidentiality, such as mandatory reporting requirements for child abuse, elder abuse, and imminent risk of harm to self or others. Clients must be informed about these limits at the beginning of the relationship.

Action Steps:

- Explain the limits of confidentiality clearly and compassionately.
- If you need to break confidentiality, inform the client about your intentions and the reasons for your actions, if possible and safe to do so.

Protecting Sensitive Information

Organizations must have policies and procedures in place to protect sensitive information, such as trauma history, mental health diagnoses, and substance use disorder treatment.

Action Steps:

- Store sensitive information securely in the electronic health record (EHR).
- Limit access to sensitive information to authorized personnel only.
- Avoid discussing sensitive information in public areas (e.g., hallways, elevators).

Confidentiality and IPV

Confidentiality is particularly critical when working with survivors of intimate partner violence (IPV). Disclosure of IPV can increase the risk of harm to the survivor if the abuser finds out

Action Steps:

- Screen for IPV in private, without the partner present.

- Use caution when documenting IPV in the medical record. Avoid using terms like "domestic violence" or "abuse" in areas of the record that the abuser might access (e.g., visit summaries, billing records).

- Use generalized language or codes to document IPV, if possible.

- Inform the client about how their information will be documented and protected.

Communicating Trauma History Sensitively in Handovers and Referrals

Communication between providers is essential for ensuring continuity of care and patient safety. However, communicating sensitive information, such as trauma history, requires careful consideration to protect the client's privacy and dignity.

Handovers

Handovers (shift changes) are a time when sensitive information is often shared between providers. It is important to conduct handovers in a way that is respectful and trauma-informed.

- **Conduct Handovers in Private:** Conduct handovers in a private setting where the conversation cannot be overheard.
- **Focus on Relevant Information:** Share only the information that is relevant to the client's current care needs. Avoid sharing unnecessary details about the trauma history.
- **Use Objective and Strengths-Based Language:** Use objective and strengths-based language when describing the client's history and behavior. Avoid judgmental or labeling language.
- **Communicate Triggers and Coping Strategies:** Share information about the client's triggers and coping strategies to help the oncoming provider provide trauma-informed care.

Example of a Trauma-Informed Handover:

"This is Maria, a 25-year-old G1P0 at 39 weeks gestation. She has a history of trauma that may impact her experience of labor. She prefers a quiet environment with minimal intrusions. She is anxious about cervical checks and prefers to decline them unless absolutely necessary. She responds well to reassurance and breathing exercises. Her partner is very supportive."

This handover provides the necessary information to the oncoming provider without sharing unnecessary details about the trauma history or using judgmental language.

Referrals

When making referrals to other providers or agencies, it is important to communicate sensitive information in a way that protects the client's confidentiality and promotes continuity of care.

- **Obtain Consent:** Obtain the client's written consent before sharing any information with the external provider or agency.
- **Share Relevant Information:** Share only the information that is necessary for the referral.
- **Use Secure Communication Channels:** Use secure communication channels (e.g., secure email, fax) to transmit sensitive information.
- **Collaborate with the Client:** Collaborate with the client on what information they want shared and how they want it shared.

The Importance of Reflection

Trauma-informed documentation and communication require ongoing reflection and practice. We must constantly examine our own biases and assumptions and strive to use language that is respectful, supportive of agency, and healing.

Action Steps:

- Review your documentation regularly to identify areas for improvement.
- Seek feedback from colleagues and clients about your communication style.
- Engage in ongoing training and education on trauma-informed care.

Moving Forward

Documentation and communication are powerful tools that can either support healing or cause further harm. By adopting trauma-informed practices in our documentation and communication, we can create a healthcare system that honors the dignity and worth of every person we care for.

In the next part of this book, we will explore how to apply the principles of trauma-informed care throughout the continuum of care, from prenatal care to postpartum support.

Key Takeaways

- Trauma-informed documentation is objective, strengths-based, and person-centered.
- Avoid judgmental and labeling language (e.g., non-compliant, difficult, resistant). Focus on behavior, not personality.
- Use "declined" instead of "refused" to honor the client's autonomy.
- Confidentiality is essential for building trust and creating safety.
- Informed consent is required for sharing information outside the healthcare team.
- Protect sensitive information securely and be mindful of confidentiality when working with IPV survivors.
- Communicate trauma history sensitively in handovers and referrals, focusing on relevant information and using objective language.

- Trauma-informed documentation and communication require ongoing reflection and practice.

Chapter 8: Trauma-Informed Prenatal Care and Birth Planning

Prenatal care is a critical opportunity to build a trusting relationship with the client, identify potential challenges, and develop a plan of care that promotes safety and agency. For trauma survivors, prenatal care can be both a source of support and a source of stress.

The frequent appointments, the invasive exams, the focus on the body, and the anticipation of birth can all be triggering. A trauma-informed approach to prenatal care recognizes these challenges and actively works to create an environment where the client feels safe, respected, and in control.

This chapter will explore strategies for building rapport and identifying triggers during routine care, discuss the process of collaborative birth planning with trauma survivors, and address common fears and anxieties related to childbirth.

Building Rapport and Identifying Triggers During Routine Care

Every interaction during prenatal care is an opportunity to build rapport and assess the client's needs. By being present, attuned, and responsive, you can create a foundation of trust that will support the client throughout their pregnancy and birth.

The First Appointment

The first prenatal appointment sets the tone for the entire relationship. It is crucial to create a welcoming and safe environment from the very beginning.

- **Warm Welcome:** Greet the client warmly and introduce yourself clearly.
- **Setting the Agenda:** Explain the purpose of the appointment and what to expect. Invite the client to share their priorities and concerns.

- **Pacing:** Go slowly and avoid rushing the conversation.
- **Inquiry about Needs:** Ask the client what they need to feel safe and comfortable during the appointment.
  - *Example:* "Is there anything I can do to make this appointment feel more comfortable for you?"

Identifying Triggers

Triggers are stimuli that remind the person of their past trauma and activate a trauma response. Triggers can be anything—a smell, a sound, a physical sensation, a tone of voice, or a situation.

During prenatal care, common triggers include:

- **Intimate Exams:** Pelvic exams, Pap smears, vaginal ultrasounds.
- **Blood Draws and IVs:** The sight of needles, the feeling of being restrained.
- **Weight Checks:** The focus on the body, the potential for judgment and shame.
- **Ultrasounds:** The vulnerability of exposure, the anxiety about the baby's well-being.
- **Questions about History:** Questions about past pregnancies, medical history, or lifestyle factors.

Recognizing Trauma Responses

Be attuned to the signs of a trauma response during prenatal appointments (as discussed in Chapter 2): hyperarousal (anxiety, agitation), hypoarousal (numbness, dissociation), and avoidance (missed appointments, difficulty making decisions).

Responding to Triggers

When you notice that a client is triggered, respond immediately to restore safety and regulation.

- **Pause the Activity:** Stop what you are doing and focus on the client.
- **Acknowledge the Distress:** Acknowledge the client's distress without judgment.
  - *Example:* "I notice you seem tense. Are you okay?"
- **Offer Support:** Offer support and reassurance.
  - *Example:* "It's okay to feel scared. I'm here with you."
- **Grounding Techniques:** Offer grounding techniques to help the client return to the present moment (e.g., deep breathing, focusing on the senses).
- **Offer Choice and Control:** Offer the client choices and control over the situation.
  - *Example:* "Do you want to take a break? We can continue later, or we can try a different approach."

Case Example The Ultrasound

Anya is having her anatomy ultrasound at 20 weeks. She has a history of sexual abuse. During the ultrasound, the technician is pressing firmly on her abdomen and talking to a colleague without acknowledging Anya. Anya becomes tense and starts holding her breath.

The midwife notices Anya's distress.

Midwife: "Anya, I notice you're holding your breath. Are you okay?"

Anya shakes her head, tears welling up in her eyes.

Midwife (to the technician): "Can you please pause for a moment?" (to Anya) "Anya, let's take a deep breath together. It's okay to feel overwhelmed. What do you need right now?"

Anya says the pressure is too much and she feels exposed.

Midwife: "Okay, thank you for telling me. (to the technician) Can you please use lighter pressure and explain what you are doing as you go? Anya, would you like me to hold your hand? We can also cover your belly more with the sheet."

By recognizing Anya's distress and intervening to restore safety and control, the midwife helps Anya regulate her nervous system and complete the ultrasound without being re-traumatized.

Collaborative Birth Planning with Trauma Survivors

Birth planning is a process of communication and collaboration between the client and the provider about the client's preferences and goals for their birth experience. For trauma survivors, birth planning is not just about choosing pain medication or birth positions. It is about creating a roadmap for safety and agency during a time of intense vulnerability.

The Goal of Trauma-Informed Birth Planning

The goal of trauma-informed birth planning is not to control every aspect of the birth (which is impossible), but to identify potential challenges and develop strategies for coping and resilience.

The Process

- **Initiate the Conversation Early:** Start the conversation about birth planning early in the pregnancy, allowing plenty of time for discussion and reflection.
- **Focus on Safety and Agency:** Frame the conversation around the client's needs for safety and agency.
  - *Example:* "Let's talk about what you need to feel safe and supported during your labor and birth."
- **Identify Triggers and Coping Strategies:** Help the client identify potential triggers during labor and birth and develop strategies for coping.
  - *Example:* "What are you most worried about? What helps you cope when you feel scared or overwhelmed?"
- **Discuss Communication Preferences:** Discuss how the client wants to communicate their needs and preferences during labor.
  - *Example:* "How will you let us know if you need a break or if something doesn't feel right?"

81

- **Develop a Plan for Interventions:** Discuss the client's preferences regarding interventions and develop a plan for shared decision-making.
- **Review and Revise:** Review and revise the birth plan throughout the pregnancy as the client's needs and preferences evolve.

Key Considerations for Trauma Survivors

When developing a birth plan with a trauma survivor, consider the following key areas:

- **Environment:** Preferences regarding lighting, sound, temperature, and privacy.
- **Support Persons:** Who the client wants present during labor and birth, and what their role will be.
- **Communication:** Preferences for communication style, language, and tone of voice.
- **Consent:** Protocols for obtaining consent for procedures and exams.
- **Intimate Exams:** Preferences regarding cervical checks (e.g., frequency, technique, alternatives).
- **Pain Management:** Preferences for pain management, including non-pharmacological and pharmacological options.
- **Interventions:** Preferences regarding interventions (e.g., induction, augmentation, episiotomy).
- **Pushing Stage:** Preferences for pushing positions and techniques.
- **Immediate Postpartum:** Preferences for immediate postpartum care, including skin-to-skin contact, cord clamping, and perineal repair.

Templates and Tools

There are many templates and tools available for trauma-informed birth planning. (See Appendix D for a sample template.) However, the most important thing is the conversation, not the document itself.

Communicating the Birth Plan

Once the birth plan is developed, it is important to communicate it clearly and effectively to the rest of the healthcare team.

- **Share the Birth Plan:** Share the birth plan with the hospital or birth center staff.
- **Advocate for the Client:** Advocate for the client's preferences and needs during labor and birth.
- **Use the Birth Plan as a Communication Tool:** Use the birth plan as a tool for communication and collaboration with the healthcare team.

Addressing Fears and Anxieties Related to Childbirth

It is normal for pregnant people to have fears and anxieties about childbirth. For trauma survivors, these fears can be intensified and overwhelming.

Common Fears and Anxieties

- Fear of pain.
- Fear of loss of control.
- Fear of re-traumatization.
- Fear of harm to self or the baby.
- Fear of judgment or mistreatment by providers.

Strategies for Addressing Fears and Anxieties

- **Validation and Normalization:** Validate the client's fears and reassure them that their feelings are normal and understandable.
- **Education and Information:** Provide the client with accurate information about the physiology of birth, pain management options, and common interventions. Knowledge supports agency.

- **Coping Skills:** Help the client develop coping skills for managing anxiety and distress during labor (e.g., breathing exercises, visualization, mindfulness).
- **Childbirth Education:** Encourage the client to attend a trauma-informed childbirth education class.
- **Therapy and Support:** Refer the client to a therapist specializing in trauma and perinatal mental health, if needed.

The Role of the Midwife

The midwife plays a crucial role in supporting the client in addressing their fears and anxieties. By providing compassionate, individualized care, the midwife can help the client develop a sense of safety, confidence, and resilience.

Conclusion

Trauma-informed prenatal care and birth planning are essential for promoting a positive and supportive birth experience for trauma survivors. By building rapport, identifying triggers, developing collaborative birth plans, and addressing fears and anxieties, we can help clients navigate the challenges of pregnancy and birth with strength and resilience.

In the next chapter, we will explore strategies for preventing birth trauma and promoting physiological birth.

Key Takeaways

- Prenatal care is a critical opportunity to build trust, identify needs, and promote safety and agency.

- Be attuned to potential triggers during routine care (e.g., exams, ultrasounds, weight checks) and respond immediately to restore safety.

- Collaborative birth planning with trauma survivors focuses on identifying triggers, developing coping strategies, and creating a roadmap for safety.

- Key considerations for trauma-informed birth planning include environment, support persons, communication, consent, and interventions.

- Address fears and anxieties related to childbirth through validation, education, coping skills development, and appropriate referrals.

- The midwife plays a crucial role in providing compassionate, individualized care that supports the client's healing and resilience.

Chapter 9: Strategies for Birth Trauma Prevention

Birth trauma is a significant public health issue with long-lasting consequences for birthing people and their families. As midwives, we have a responsibility to actively work to prevent birth trauma and promote positive birth experiences.

Birth trauma prevention starts long before labor begins. It is rooted in the principles of trauma-informed care: safety, trustworthiness, collaboration, agency, and choice.

This chapter will explore evidence-based strategies for birth trauma prevention, including continuity of care models, trauma-informed approaches to pain management, minimizing unnecessary interventions, addressing obstetric violence, and communication protocols during emergencies.

Continuity of Care Models

Continuity of care models, particularly midwifery-led continuity of care, have been shown to improve birth outcomes and reduce the risk of birth trauma (Sandall et al., 2016).

What is Continuity of Care?

Continuity of care means that the birthing person receives care from the same provider or small team of providers throughout their pregnancy, labor, birth, and postpartum period.

Benefits of Continuity of Care

- **Trusting Relationships:** Continuity of care allows for the development of a trusting relationship between the client and the provider. This relationship is the foundation of safety and support during labor and birth.

- **Individualized Care:** When providers know their clients well, they can provide individualized care that is tailored to their specific needs, preferences, and goals.
- **Improved Communication:** Continuity of care improves communication and collaboration between the client and the provider.
- **Increased Agency:** Clients who receive continuity of care often feel more supported in their agency and in control of their birth experience.
- **Reduced Interventions:** Continuity of care is associated with lower rates of interventions, such as epidurals, episiotomies, and Cesarean sections.

Implementing Continuity of Care

Implementing continuity of care models requires systemic changes in how maternity care is organized and delivered.

- **Midwifery Group Practices:** Midwifery group practices provide care by a small team of midwives who share a caseload and provide 24/7 coverage for labor and birth.
- **Caseload Midwifery:** Caseload midwifery involves a single midwife providing care to a small number of clients throughout their perinatal journey.
- **Community-Based Care:** Community-based midwifery models provide care in the community setting, often serving marginalized populations.

Trauma-Informed Approaches to Pain Management

Pain management is a critical aspect of the birth experience. For trauma survivors, pain can be particularly triggering and overwhelming. A trauma-informed approach to pain management recognizes the complex interplay between pain, fear, and trauma, and prioritizes the client's comfort, control, and autonomy.

The Fear-Tension-Pain Cycle

As discussed in Chapter 2, fear and stress can increase the perception of pain, leading to the fear-tension-pain cycle. Trauma-informed pain management focuses on breaking this cycle by addressing the underlying fear and promoting relaxation and coping.

Non-Pharmacological Pain Management

Non-pharmacological pain management strategies can be highly effective in reducing pain and promoting comfort during labor. They also enhance the client's sense of control and agency.

- **Continuous Labor Support:** Continuous support by a trained doula or supportive partner can significantly reduce pain perception and the need for medication.
- **Movement and Positioning:** Encouraging movement and upright positioning can help labor progress and reduce pain.
- **Hydrotherapy:** Warm water immersion (e.g., shower or bath) can promote relaxation and reduce pain.
- **Breathing and Relaxation Techniques:** Deep breathing, visualization, and mindfulness techniques can help the client cope with contractions and stay grounded.
- **Massage and Touch:** Massage and counter-pressure can help relieve muscle tension and pain.

Pharmacological Pain Management

Pharmacological pain management options, such as nitrous oxide and epidurals, can also be helpful for managing pain during labor. A trauma-informed approach to pharmacological pain management ensures that the client has the information and support they need to make informed choices about their pain relief.

- **Informed Consent:** Provide clear, balanced information about the benefits, risks, and alternatives of pharmacological pain management options.
- **Respect for Choice:** Respect the client's choice to use or decline pain medication, without judgment or coercion.

- **Timing and Pacing:** Administer pain medication at the client's request and pace the administration to maximize comfort and control.
- **Addressing Fears and Concerns:** Address any fears or concerns the client may have about pain medication (e.g., fear of needles, fear of loss of control).

Epidurals and Trauma Survivors

Epidurals can be particularly challenging for trauma survivors. The feeling of numbness, the loss of mobility, and the need for invasive procedures (e.g., urinary catheterization) can be triggering.

- **Trauma-Informed Epidural Placement:**
  - Explain the procedure clearly and obtain explicit consent.
  - Provide continuous support and reassurance during the procedure.
  - Offer choices and control whenever possible (e.g., positioning, timing).
  - Minimize exposure and maximize privacy.
- **Managing Side Effects:**
  - Address the client's concerns about numbness and loss of mobility.
  - Use intermittent urinary catheterization instead of continuous indwelling catheters, if possible.
  - Encourage position changes and movement as much as possible.

Minimizing Unnecessary Interventions and Addressing Obstetric Violence

Unnecessary interventions during labor and birth can increase the risk of complications and trauma. Obstetric violence, which includes any form of mistreatment, disrespect, or abuse during childbirth, is a violation of human rights and a major cause of birth trauma.

Minimizing Unnecessary Interventions

- **Promoting Physiological Birth:** Support the physiological process of birth by creating a safe, supportive environment that promotes oxytocin release and minimizes stress.
- **Evidence-Based Practice:** Use evidence-based practices to guide clinical decision-making and avoid routine interventions that are not supported by evidence (e.g., routine episiotomies, routine continuous fetal monitoring for low-risk pregnancies).
- **Shared Decision-Making:** Engage in shared decision-making with the client about all interventions, ensuring they have the information and support they need to make informed choices.
- **Patience and Watchful Waiting:** Practice patience and watchful waiting, allowing labor to unfold at its own pace as long as the birthing person and the baby are safe.

Addressing Obstetric Violence

Obstetric violence is a systemic issue that requires a systemic response. As midwives, we have a responsibility to recognize and address obstetric violence in our practice and in the system.

- **Zero Tolerance Policy:** Advocate for and enforce a zero-tolerance policy for obstetric violence in your workplace.
- **Respectful Maternity Care:** Provide respectful maternity care that honors the dignity, autonomy, and preferences of every birthing person.
- **Informed Consent:** Ensure that all procedures and treatments are performed with the client's informed consent.
- **Accountability:** Hold yourself and your colleagues accountable for providing respectful and compassionate care.
- **Advocacy:** Advocate for policies and practices that promote human rights in childbirth.

Communication Protocols During Emergencies

Emergencies during labor and birth can be terrifying and chaotic. The way we communicate during emergencies can significantly impact the client's experience and their risk of trauma.

Trauma-Informed Communication During Emergencies

- **Clear and Calm Communication:** Communicate clearly and calmly, even in high-stress situations. Avoid shouting or using alarming language.
- **Explain What Is Happening:** Explain what is happening and why, using simple, accessible language.
- **Maintain Connection:** Maintain connection with the client throughout the emergency. Make eye contact, use touch respectfully, and offer reassurance.
- **Designated Communicator:** Assign a designated communicator to provide continuous updates and support to the client and their family.
- **Debriefing:** After the emergency is resolved, debrief the experience with the client and their family. Answer questions, validate their feelings, and offer support.

Case Example The Shoulder Dystocia

A shoulder dystocia is an obstetric emergency that requires immediate intervention. Here's how to apply trauma-informed communication protocols in this scenario:

- **Clear Communication:** The midwife recognizes the shoulder dystocia and calls for help calmly and clearly. "I have a shoulder dystocia. I need assistance."
- **Explanation:** The midwife explains to the client what is happening and what needs to be done. "The baby's shoulder is stuck. I need you to stop pushing and change position so we can help the baby out."
- **Narration:** The midwife narrates her actions as she performs the maneuvers to resolve the dystocia. "I'm going to press on your belly now." "Now I'm going to help the baby's arm out."

91

- **Reassurance:** The midwife offers reassurance throughout the process. "You are doing great. We are taking good care of you and your baby."
- **Debriefing:** After the baby is born, the midwife debriefs the experience with the client and their family. "That was scary. I want to explain what happened and answer any questions you have."

Conclusion

Birth trauma prevention is an essential aspect of trauma-informed midwifery care. By implementing continuity of care models, using trauma-informed approaches to pain management, minimizing unnecessary interventions, addressing obstetric violence, and communicating effectively during emergencies, we can create a maternity care system where every birthing person feels safe, respected, and supported in their agency.

In the next chapter, we will explore strategies for managing triggered responses during labor and supporting clients who become dysregulated.

Key Takeaways

- Birth trauma prevention is rooted in the principles of trauma-informed care: safety, trustworthiness, collaboration, agency, and choice.

- Continuity of care models improve birth outcomes and reduce the risk of birth trauma by fostering trusting relationships and individualized care.

- Trauma-informed pain management prioritizes the client's comfort, control, and autonomy, utilizing both non-pharmacological and pharmacological strategies.

- Minimizing unnecessary interventions and addressing obstetric violence are essential for preventing birth trauma and promoting human rights in childbirth.

- Communication protocols during emergencies should prioritize clear, calm communication, connection, and debriefing.

Chapter 10: Managing Triggered Responses During Labor

Labor is an intense, vulnerable experience. For trauma survivors, the physical sensations, the loss of control, and the presence of medical providers can be deeply triggering. No matter how much preparation and planning you do, it is likely that a trauma survivor will experience triggered responses during labor.

Your ability to recognize and respond effectively to these responses is crucial for preventing re-traumatization and promoting a positive birth experience. This is where your understanding of the neurobiology of trauma (Chapter 2) becomes essential.

This chapter will focus on identifying dissociation, flashbacks, and panic in the birthing room, and provide immediate response protocols for helping clients get grounded, regulated, and reconnected. We will also discuss how to support partners and support persons during client activation.

Identifying Dissociation, Flashbacks, and Panic in the Birthing Room

The first step in managing a triggered response is recognizing that it is happening. As we discussed in Chapter 2, trauma responses can manifest in various ways, including hyperarousal (fight or flight) and hypoarousal (freeze or shutdown).

Dissociation

Dissociation is a state of disconnection from the present moment, the body, or the self. It is a common response to overwhelming stress or trauma. During labor, dissociation can look like:

- **Spacing Out:** The client may seem distant, "not there," or have a glazed look in their eyes.

- **Numbness:** The client may report feeling numb, floaty, or disconnected from their body.
- **Difficulty Responding:** The client may have difficulty responding to questions or following instructions.
- **Memory Gaps:** The client may have gaps in their memory of the labor process.
- **Out-of-Body Experience:** The client may report feeling like they are watching themselves from outside their body.

Dissociation is a protective mechanism. It allows the mind to escape a situation that feels unbearable. However, during labor, dissociation can interfere with the physiological process of birth and the client's ability to connect with their baby.

Flashbacks

A *flashback* is an intrusive memory of a past trauma that feels like it is happening in the present moment. Flashbacks can be visual, auditory, olfactory, or somatic (physical sensations). During labor, flashbacks can be triggered by physical sensations (e.g., pain, pressure), procedures (e.g., cervical exams), or environmental cues (e.g., smells, sounds).

Flashbacks can look like:

- **Sudden Change in Behavior:** The client may suddenly become agitated, fearful, or withdrawn.
- **Intense Emotional Reaction:** The client may experience intense emotions that seem disproportionate to the situation.
- **Sensory Experiences:** The client may report seeing images, hearing sounds, or smelling odors related to the trauma.
- **Physical Sensations:** The client may experience physical sensations related to the trauma (e.g., pain, choking).
- **Loss of Orientation:** The client may seem confused or disoriented to time and place.

Panic

Panic is a state of intense fear and anxiety, accompanied by physical symptoms such as racing heart, shortness of breath, dizziness, and trembling. Panic is a hyperarousal response (fight or flight). During labor, panic can be triggered by pain, loss of control, or fear for safety.

Panic can look like:

- **Agitation and Restlessness:** The client may seem unable to get comfortable, thrashing, or trying to get out of bed.
- **Rapid Breathing or Hyperventilation:** The client may be breathing rapidly and shallowly.
- **Expressions of Terror:** The client may express feeling terrified, overwhelmed, or like they are going to die.
- **Inability to Cope:** The client may seem unable to cope with the contractions and may be pleading for help.

Immediate Response Protocols

When a client is triggered during labor, your immediate response should focus on restoring safety, regulation, and connection. Remember, you cannot reason with a person whose thinking brain is offline. You must address the physiological response first.

The Three R's of Responding to Triggers

1. **Recognize:** Recognize the signs of a trauma response.
2. **Respond:** Respond immediately to restore safety and regulation.
3. **Resist Re-traumatization:** Avoid actions that may escalate the distress or cause further harm.

General Principles for Responding to Triggers

- **Stay Calm:** Maintain a calm, regulated presence. Your calm nervous system can help regulate the client's nervous system (co-regulation).

- **Create Safety:** Create a safe environment by minimizing stimulation (e.g., dimming the lights, reducing noise) and ensuring privacy.
- **Connect:** Connect with the client through eye contact (if comfortable), gentle touch (if consented), and a calm voice.
- **Validate:** Validate the client's feelings and experiences without judgment.
- **Support Agency:** Offer the client choices and control over the situation.

Grounding Techniques

Grounding techniques are strategies for helping the client return to the present moment and reconnect with their body and surroundings. They are particularly helpful for managing dissociation and flashbacks.

- **Sensory Grounding (5-4-3-2-1 Technique):** Ask the client to identify 5 things they can see, 4 things they can touch, 3 things they can hear, 2 things they can smell, and 1 thing they can taste.
- **Physical Grounding:** Encourage the client to focus on physical sensations in their body.
  - *Example:* "Press your feet into the floor." "Squeeze my hand."
- **Movement:** Encourage gentle movement, such as rocking, swaying, or stretching.
- **Temperature Change:** Use temperature changes to bring the client back to the present moment (e.g., holding an ice cube, splashing cold water on the face).
- **Orienting to the Present:** Remind the client where they are and what is happening.
  - *Example:* "You are safe. You are in the hospital. You are having a baby. I am here with you."

Co-Regulation

Co-regulation involves using your own regulated nervous system to help the client regulate their nervous system.

- **Breathing Together:** Invite the client to breathe with you. Use slow, deep breaths.
- **Calm Voice:** Speak in a calm, soothing voice.
- **Attuned Touch:** Offer attuned touch, such as holding the client's hand or placing a hand on their shoulder (if consented).
- **Mirroring:** Mirror the client's emotions with compassion and empathy.

Re-establishing Safety

- **Address the Trigger:** If possible, identify and address the trigger that caused the response.
- **Modify the Environment:** Modify the environment to promote safety and comfort.
- **Adjust the Plan of Care:** Adjust the plan of care to meet the client's needs and preferences.

Specific Protocols for Different Responses

Responding to Dissociation (Hypoarousal)

When a client is dissociated, the goal is to gently bring them back to the present moment and reconnect them with their body.

- **Use a Calm, Gentle Voice:** Speak softly and gently.
- **Orient to the Present:** Remind the client where they are and what is happening.
- **Use Sensory Grounding:** Use sensory grounding techniques, focusing on touch, smell, and sound.
- **Encourage Movement:** Encourage gentle movement to help the client reconnect with their body.
- **Avoid Sudden Movements or Loud Noises:** Avoid actions that may startle or overwhelm the client.

Responding to Flashbacks and Panic (Hyperarousal)

When a client is experiencing a flashback or panic, the goal is to help them feel safe, grounded, and in control.

- **Create Safety:** Create a safe environment by minimizing stimulation and ensuring privacy.
- **Use a Calm, Firm Voice:** Speak clearly and confidently.
- **Orient to the Present:** Remind the client that they are safe and that the trauma is not happening now.
- **Use Physical Grounding:** Use physical grounding techniques, focusing on movement, temperature change, and deep pressure.
- **Breathing Techniques:** Encourage slow, deep breaths to help regulate the nervous system.
- **Agency:** Offer choices and control over the situation.

What NOT to Do When a Client Is Triggered

- **Do not panic or become reactive.**
- **Do not judge or criticize the client's response.**
- **Do not try to reason with the client or force them to talk about the trauma.**
- **Do not touch the client without permission.**
- **Do not abandon the client.**

Case Example Managing a Flashback During Labor

Tanya is in active labor. During a cervical check, she suddenly becomes agitated and starts yelling, "Get off me! Don't touch me!" Her eyes are wide with fear, and she is trying to push the midwife away.

The midwife recognizes this as a flashback.

Midwife (calmly and firmly): "Tanya, I am stopping the exam. I am removing my hands now. You are safe." (Creating safety)

The midwife moves back slightly to give Tanya space, but stays close enough to offer support.

Midwife: "Tanya, look at me. It's me, your midwife. You are in the hospital. You are having a baby. That was a memory. It is not happening now." (Orienting to the present)

The midwife invites Tanya to use a grounding technique.

Midwife: "Tanya, can you press your feet into the bed? Feel the sheets under your legs. Take a deep breath with me." (Grounding)

Tanya gradually starts to calm down.

Midwife: "You did great. That was scary. What do you need right now to feel safe?" (Validation, supporting agency)

Supporting Partners and Support Persons During Client Activation

Witnessing a loved one experiencing a triggered response can be distressing and overwhelming for partners and support persons. They may feel helpless, scared, or confused. Supporting the partner is an essential part of trauma-informed care.

Before Labor

- **Education:** Provide education to the partner about trauma, triggers, and trauma responses during labor.
- **Preparation:** Help the partner develop strategies for supporting the client during labor, including grounding techniques and advocacy skills.
- **Communication:** Encourage the partner to communicate with the client about their needs and preferences for support.

During Labor

- **Acknowledge Distress:** Acknowledge the partner's distress and validate their feelings.
- **Provide Information:** Explain what is happening and what you are doing to support the client.
- **Offer Guidance:** Offer guidance on how the partner can support the client (e.g., breathing together, offering touch, advocating for the client's needs).

- **Offer Breaks:** Encourage the partner to take breaks and care for themselves.

After the Triggered Response

- **Debrief the Experience:** Debrief the experience with the partner and offer support.
- **Provide Resources:** Provide the partner with resources for their own support, if needed (e.g., therapy, support groups).

Conclusion

Managing triggered responses during labor is a critical skill for trauma-informed midwives. By recognizing the signs of dissociation, flashbacks, and panic, and responding effectively with grounding techniques, co-regulation, and re-establishment of safety, we can help clients navigate the challenges of labor without being re-traumatized. Supporting partners and support persons is also essential for creating a safe and supportive birth environment.

In the next chapter, we will explore trauma-informed care in the postpartum period, including postpartum PTSD support and infant feeding support.

Key Takeaways

- Triggered responses during labor are common for trauma survivors and require immediate attention.

- Identify the signs of dissociation (spacing out, numbness), flashbacks (intrusive memories, intense emotions), and panic (fear, agitation).

- The immediate response should focus on restoring safety, regulation, and connection (The Three R's: Recognize, Respond, Resist Re-traumatization).

- Grounding techniques help the client return to the present moment and reconnect with their body.

- Co-regulation involves using your own regulated nervous system to help the client regulate their nervous system.

- Specific protocols for responding to hypoarousal (dissociation) and hyperarousal (flashbacks, panic) focus on gentle grounding and re-establishment of safety.

- Supporting partners and support persons is essential for creating a safe and supportive birth environment.

Chapter 11: Postpartum Care and PTSD Support

The postpartum period is a time of significant transition and vulnerability. For trauma survivors, this period can be particularly challenging. The physical recovery from birth, the hormonal shifts, the demands of newborn care, and the potential for postpartum mood disorders can all exacerbate the effects of trauma.

A trauma-informed approach to postpartum care recognizes these challenges and provides sensitive, individualized support that promotes healing and resilience.

This chapter will explore trauma-informed care in the immediate postpartum period, discuss screening and assessment for postpartum PTSD, address the unique challenges of infant feeding support for trauma survivors, and emphasize the importance of debriefing the birth experience.

The Immediate Postpartum Trauma-Informed Perineal Repair and Protecting the "Golden Hour"

The immediate postpartum period (the first few hours after birth) is a critical time for bonding, rest, and recovery. A trauma-informed approach to this period prioritizes the physical and emotional safety of the birthing person and the baby.

Trauma-Informed Perineal Repair

Perineal repair can be a vulnerable and triggering experience for trauma survivors, particularly those with a history of sexual abuse or a traumatic birth experience.

- **Informed Consent:** Obtain explicit informed consent before performing the repair. Explain the procedure clearly and discuss pain management options.

- **Adequate Anesthesia:** Ensure adequate anesthesia before starting the repair. Check in frequently with the client about their comfort level.
- **Privacy and Respect:** Ensure privacy and minimize exposure. Treat the client with respect and dignity.
- **Narration and Pacing:** Narrate your actions step-by-step and go slowly.
- **Choice and Control:** Offer the client choices and control over the procedure (e.g., positioning, timing).
- **Support and Reassurance:** Provide continuous support and reassurance throughout the procedure.

Protecting the "Golden Hour"

The "golden hour" (the first hour after birth) is a crucial time for bonding and the initiation of breastfeeding/chestfeeding. Protecting this time from unnecessary interruptions and interventions is essential for promoting a positive postpartum experience.

- **Skin-to-Skin Contact:** Facilitate immediate and uninterrupted skin-to-skin contact between the birthing person and the baby.
- **Delayed Procedures:** Delay routine procedures (e.g., weighing the baby, administering vitamin K) until after the first hour, if possible and safe to do so.
- **Quiet and Calm Environment:** Create a quiet, calm environment that supports bonding and rest.
- **Minimal Intrusions:** Minimize intrusions by staff and visitors.
- **Support for Feeding:** Provide gentle, supportive assistance with the initiation of feeding, respecting the client's choices and preferences.

Screening and Assessment for Postpartum PTSD

Postpartum PTSD (P-PTSD) is a serious mental health condition that affects 3% to 16% of birthing people (Grekin & O'Hara, 2014). Early identification and treatment of P-PTSD are crucial for the well-being of the birthing person and the family.

Risk Factors for P-PTSD

- History of trauma (especially sexual abuse or assault).
- Previous history of mental health conditions (e.g., depression, anxiety, PTSD).
- Traumatic birth experience (e.g., emergency C-section, severe complications, feeling unsupported or mistreated).
- Lack of social support.
- Infant admission to the NICU.

Screening for P-PTSD

Routine screening for P-PTSD should be conducted during the postpartum period.

- **Timing:** Screening should be conducted at multiple time points during the first year postpartum (e.g., at the postpartum visit, at well-child visits).
- **Tools:** Use validated screening tools, such as the Perinatal PTSD Questionnaire (PPQ) or the PTSD Checklist for DSM-5 (PCL-5).
- **Trauma-Informed Approach:** Conduct screening in a trauma-informed way, ensuring safety, confidentiality, and informed consent.

Differentiating P-PTSD from PPD/PPA

P-PTSD often co-occurs with postpartum depression (PPD) and postpartum anxiety (PPA), and the symptoms can overlap. However, there are some key differences.

- **PPD:** Characterized by persistent sadness, hopelessness, loss of interest in activities, changes in sleep and appetite, and difficulty bonding with the baby.
- **PPA:** Characterized by excessive worry, anxiety, panic attacks, and obsessive thoughts.

- **P-PTSD:** Characterized by symptoms related to the traumatic birth experience, including intrusive memories, flashbacks, nightmares, avoidance of reminders of the birth, hyperarousal (irritability, anxiety, hypervigilance), and negative changes in mood and cognition.

Assessment and Referral

If a client screens positive for P-PTSD, a comprehensive assessment should be conducted to confirm the diagnosis and determine the appropriate level of care.

- **Clinical Interview:** Conduct a clinical interview to explore the client's symptoms, history, and functioning.
- **Referral:** Refer the client to a mental health professional specializing in trauma and perinatal mental health for further evaluation and treatment.
- **Trauma-Specific Treatment:** Treatment for P-PTSD often involves trauma-specific therapies, such as Eye Movement Desensitization and Reprocessing (EMDR) or Trauma-Focused Cognitive Behavioral Therapy (TF-CBT).

Infant Feeding Support for Trauma Survivors

Infant feeding can be a major challenge for trauma survivors. A trauma-informed approach to infant feeding support prioritizes the mental health and autonomy of the birthing person over the method of feeding.

Challenges for Trauma Survivors

- **Triggers:** Breastfeeding/chestfeeding can be triggering for survivors of sexual abuse due to the physical sensation, the feeling of being "touched out," or the association with the abuse.
- **Pain and Discomfort:** Trauma survivors may experience increased pain or discomfort during feeding due to hyperarousal or dissociation.

- **Shame and Guilt:** Trauma survivors may feel shame or guilt if they struggle with feeding, feeling like their body is failing them.
- **Pressure to Breastfeed:** The pressure to breastfeed from providers and society can be overwhelming and undermine agency.

Trauma-Informed Feeding Support

- **Respect for Choice:** Respect the client's choice of feeding method (breastfeeding/chestfeeding, formula feeding, or combination feeding) without judgment or coercion.
- **Validation and Normalization:** Validate the client's feelings and experiences related to feeding and normalize their challenges.
- **Focus on Mental Health:** Prioritize the client's mental health and well-being. A healthy parent is more important than the method of feeding.
- **Agency and Control:** Support the client to make decisions about feeding that feel right for them.
- **Practical Strategies:** Offer practical strategies for making feeding feel safe and manageable.
  - *Example:* Adjusting positioning to minimize exposure, using grounding techniques during feeding, taking breaks when needed.
- **Referral:** Refer the client to a lactation consultant or therapist with expertise in trauma-informed feeding support, if needed.

Debriefing the Birth Experience Validation and Follow-up

Debriefing the birth experience is an essential part of trauma-informed postpartum care. It provides an opportunity for the client to process their experience, ask questions, and receive validation and support.

The Goal of Debriefing

The goal of debriefing is not to analyze the clinical details of the birth, but to explore the client's subjective experience and emotional response to the birth.

Timing of Debriefing

Debriefing should be offered at multiple time points during the postpartum period.

- **Immediate Postpartum:** A brief check-in in the immediate postpartum period to acknowledge the birth experience and offer support.
- **Postpartum Visit:** A more in-depth debriefing at the postpartum visit (e.g., at 2-6 weeks postpartum).
- **Ongoing Support:** Ongoing opportunities for debriefing and support throughout the first year postpartum.

Strategies for Trauma-Informed Debriefing

- **Invite the Conversation:** Invite the client to share their birth story in their own words.
  - *Example:* "How would you describe your birth experience? What stands out to you the most?"
- **Active Listening:** Listen actively and reflectively, without interruption or judgment.
- **Validation:** Validate the client's feelings and experiences, even if they differ from your perception of the birth.
- **Clarification:** Answer the client's questions and clarify any misunderstandings about the birth events.
- **Apology:** If appropriate, offer a genuine apology for any actions or interactions that caused distress or harm.
- **Follow-up:** Follow up with the client about any concerns or needs identified during the debriefing.

Case Example Debriefing a Traumatic Birth

Sarah had a traumatic birth experience involving an emergency C-section. At her postpartum visit, the midwife invites her to debrief the experience.

Midwife: "Sarah, I know your birth experience was not what you had planned. I want to offer you a space to talk about it, if you would like to. How are you feeling about it?"

Sarah shares that she felt terrified and helpless during the C-section and is struggling with flashbacks and nightmares.

Midwife: "Sarah, that sounds incredibly difficult. It makes sense that you would feel terrified and helpless. It was a scary situation. (Validation) I'm so sorry that you had that experience. (Compassion)

"What stands out to you the most about the experience? Are there any parts that you would like to talk about or ask questions about?" (Exploration)

The midwife answers Sarah's questions about the clinical details of the C-section and reassures her that she did nothing wrong.

Midwife: "It sounds like you are struggling with flashbacks and nightmares. These are common responses to a traumatic experience. (Normalization) I want you to know that help is available. I can refer you to a therapist who specializes in birth trauma, if you are interested." (Referral)

Conclusion

Trauma-informed postpartum care is essential for promoting healing and resilience in trauma survivors. By providing sensitive, individualized support during the immediate postpartum period, screening and assessing for P-PTSD, offering trauma-informed feeding support, and debriefing the birth experience, we can help clients navigate the challenges of the postpartum period and thrive as new parents.

In the next part of the book, we will explore specific challenges and populations in trauma-informed midwifery care, including caring for abuse survivors and marginalized communities.

Key Takeaways

- The postpartum period is a time of vulnerability for trauma survivors, requiring sensitive, individualized support.
- Trauma-informed perineal repair prioritizes consent, comfort, and control.
- Protecting the "golden hour" promotes bonding and rest and minimizes unnecessary interruptions.
- Screening and assessment for postpartum PTSD (P-PTSD) are crucial for early identification and treatment.
- P-PTSD symptoms include intrusive memories, flashbacks, avoidance, hyperarousal, and negative changes in mood and cognition.
- Trauma-informed feeding support prioritizes the mental health and autonomy of the birthing person over the method of feeding.
- Debriefing the birth experience provides an opportunity for validation, clarification, and support.

Chapter 12: Specific Protocols for Abuse Survivors

While the principles of trauma-informed care apply to all clients, survivors of abuse (including sexual abuse, physical abuse, and intimate partner violence) often have specific needs and challenges during the perinatal period.

This chapter will provide specific protocols for caring for survivors of sexual abuse and assault, addressing common triggers related to intimate exams and procedures, and strategies for minimizing re-traumatization. We will also discuss protocols for caring for survivors of intimate partner violence (IPV), including safety planning.

Caring for Survivors of Sexual Abuse and Assault

Survivors of sexual abuse and assault often experience heightened vulnerability and anxiety during pregnancy and birth. The physical sensations, the loss of control, and the power dynamics in the healthcare setting can all be triggering.

Understanding the Impact of Sexual Abuse

Sexual abuse can have long-lasting effects on a person's sense of safety, body image, sexuality, and relationships. Survivors may struggle with:

- Difficulty trusting others, especially those in positions of authority.
- Fear of loss of control.
- Negative body image and disconnection from the body.
- Pain or discomfort during sexual activity or intimate exams.
- Flashbacks, dissociation, or panic attacks during stressful situations.

Trauma-Informed Care for Sexual Abuse Survivors

- **Sensitive Inquiry:** Ask about a history of sexual abuse in a sensitive and trauma-informed way (as discussed in Chapter 5).
- **Validation and Normalization:** Validate the survivor's feelings and experiences and normalize their responses to the perinatal period.
- **Agency and Control:** Prioritize the survivor's agency and control throughout the care process.
- **Informed Consent:** Ensure explicit informed consent for all procedures and exams.
- **Trigger Identification:** Help the survivor identify potential triggers during pregnancy and birth and develop coping strategies.
- **Referral:** Refer the survivor to a therapist or support group specializing in sexual abuse recovery, if needed.

Specific Triggers Related to Cervical Exams, Pushing, and Exposure

Intimate exams, the pushing stage of labor, and exposure of the body can be particularly triggering for sexual abuse survivors.

Cervical Exams

- **Minimize Frequency:** Minimize the frequency of cervical exams, performing them only when clinically necessary.
- **Trauma-Informed Techniques:** Use trauma-informed techniques during cervical exams (as discussed in Chapter 6), such as using adequate lubrication, going slowly, and establishing a stop signal.
- **Alternative Positions:** Offer alternative positions for cervical exams (e.g., side-lying, semi-sitting) that may feel less vulnerable.
- **Self-Insertion:** Offer the option of self-insertion of the speculum or ultrasound probe, if applicable.
-

Pushing Stage

The pushing stage of labor can be intense and overwhelming. The physical sensations of pressure and stretching, the feeling of the body opening, and the presence of providers between the legs can trigger flashbacks or dissociation.

- **Avoid Coached Pushing:** Avoid directed or coached pushing (e.g., "hold your breath and push as hard as you can"). Encourage the survivor to push instinctively and follow their body's urges.
- **Upright Positions:** Encourage upright pushing positions (e.g., squatting, hands and knees) that promote a sense of control and agency.
- **Minimize Exposure:** Minimize exposure of the genitals during the pushing stage.
- **Supportive Language:** Use supportive and encouraging language, avoiding phrases that may be triggering (e.g., "open up," "relax").

Exposure

Exposure of the body can be deeply distressing for sexual abuse survivors.

- **Maximize Privacy:** Ensure privacy during appointments and procedures.
- **Minimize Exposure:** Use draping techniques to minimize exposure of the body.
- **Offer Choices:** Offer the client choices about what to wear during labor and birth.
- **Ask for Permission:** Ask for permission before uncovering the client's body.

Protocols to Minimize Re-traumatization During Procedures

Procedures such as IV insertion, epidural placement, and perineal repair can also be triggering for sexual abuse survivors.

- **Clear Explanation:** Explain the procedure clearly and obtain explicit consent.
- **Continuous Support:** Provide continuous support and reassurance during the procedure.
- **Grounding Techniques:** Use grounding techniques to help the survivor stay present and regulated.
- **Pain Management:** Ensure adequate pain management during procedures.
- **Pacing and Control:** Go slowly and offer the client choices and control over the procedure whenever possible.

Caring for Survivors of Intimate Partner Violence (IPV) Safety Planning

Intimate partner violence (IPV) is a serious issue that requires a sensitive and strategic response. The primary goal when caring for IPV survivors is to promote their safety and autonomy.

Recognizing the Signs of IPV

Be aware of the signs of IPV, which can be subtle or overt.

- **Physical Signs:** Unexplained injuries, bruises in various stages of healing.
- **Behavioral Signs:** Missed appointments, late arrival, seeming fearful or evasive, difficulty making decisions.
- **Partner Behavior:** Partner who is overly controlling, refuses to leave the room, answers questions for the client, or is verbally abusive.

Screening for IPV

Routine screening for IPV should be conducted during the perinatal period.

- **Private Setting:** Screen for IPV in a private setting, without the partner present.

- **Trauma-Informed Approach:** Use a trauma-informed approach to screening (as discussed in Chapter 5), ensuring safety, confidentiality, and informed consent.
- **Direct Questions:** Ask direct questions about the client's safety and experiences of violence.

Responding to Disclosures of IPV

If a client discloses IPV, respond with compassion, validation, and support.

- **Believe the Survivor:** Believe the survivor's story and validate their feelings.
- **Assess Immediate Safety:** Assess the survivor's immediate safety and risk of harm.
- **Offer Resources and Referrals:** Offer resources and referrals for domestic violence support services (e.g., shelters, hotlines, legal aid).
- **Respect Autonomy:** Respect the survivor's autonomy and right to make decisions about their own life. Avoid telling the survivor what to do or pressuring them to leave the relationship.

Safety Planning

Safety planning is a process of identifying strategies for staying safe in an abusive relationship or planning to leave safely.

- **Collaborative Process:** Safety planning should be a collaborative process between the provider and the survivor.
- **Individualized Plan:** The safety plan should be individualized to the survivor's specific needs and circumstances.
- **Key Components of a Safety Plan:**
  - Identifying safe places to go in an emergency.
  - Packing an emergency bag with important documents, keys, and money.
  - Establishing a code word or signal to alert friends or family if in danger.

o   Strategies for protecting children.

o   Strategies for staying safe online and protecting privacy.

Documentation of IPV

Documentation of IPV requires careful consideration to protect the survivor's safety and confidentiality (as discussed in Chapter 7).

- **Objective Language:** Use objective language and quote the survivor directly, if possible.
- **Avoid Judgmental Language:** Avoid judgmental or blaming language.
- **Secure Storage:** Store documentation securely and limit access to authorized personnel.

Conclusion

Caring for abuse survivors requires sensitivity, skill, and a commitment to prioritizing safety and agency. By implementing specific protocols for minimizing re-traumatization during intimate exams and procedures, and by providing compassionate and strategic support for IPV survivors, we can help survivors navigate the challenges of the perinatal period and promote healing and resilience.

In the next chapter, we will explore the intersectionality of trauma, cultural humility, and systemic oppression in midwifery care.

Key Takeaways

- Survivors of abuse have specific needs and challenges during the perinatal period that require a trauma-informed approach.
- Cervical exams, the pushing stage, and exposure of the body can be particularly triggering for sexual abuse survivors.
- Protocols for minimizing re-traumatization include minimizing frequency of exams, using trauma-informed techniques, offering alternative positions, and maximizing privacy.

- The primary goal when caring for IPV survivors is to promote their safety and autonomy.

- Safety planning is a collaborative process of identifying strategies for staying safe in an abusive relationship or planning to leave safely.

- Documentation of IPV requires careful consideration to protect the survivor's safety and confidentiality.

Chapter 13: Intersectionality, Cultural Humility, and Systemic Trauma

Trauma does not exist in a vacuum. It is shaped by the social, cultural, and political context in which it occurs. A trauma-informed approach to midwifery care must recognize the intersectionality of trauma with other identities and experiences, and actively address the impact of systemic oppression and historical trauma.

This chapter will explore the concepts of intersectionality, cultural humility, and systemic trauma, and provide strategies for providing culturally safe and anti-racist care. We will also discuss the specific needs of LGBTQIA+ birthing people.

Recognizing Historical and Racial Trauma in Maternity Care

As discussed in Chapter 1, historical trauma and racial trauma have a significant impact on the health and well-being of Black, Indigenous, and other People of Color (BIPOC).

Historical Trauma

Historical trauma refers to the cumulative emotional and psychological wounding across generations, stemming from massive group trauma experiences (e.g., slavery, genocide, colonization, forced displacement).

In the context of maternity care, historical trauma can manifest as:

- **Distrust of the Healthcare System:** A deep and justified distrust of the healthcare system due to a history of medical abuse and exploitation.
- **Fear of Harm:** A fear of being harmed, mistreated, or discriminated against by providers.
- **Heightened Stress Response:** A heightened stress response due to the cumulative impact of intergenerational trauma.

Racial Trauma

Racial trauma refers to the mental and emotional injury caused by encounters with racial bias, discrimination, and violence.

In the context of maternity care, racial trauma can manifest as:

- **Weathering:** The cumulative impact of chronic stress from living in a racist society, leading to premature aging and poorer health outcomes (Geronimus et al., 2006).
- **Hypervigilance:** A state of constant alertness and vigilance for potential threats of discrimination or harm.
- **Internalized Racism:** The internalization of negative stereotypes and beliefs about one's own racial group.

The Impact of Racism and Discrimination on Outcomes

The impact of racism and discrimination on maternal and infant health outcomes is undeniable. As discussed in Chapter 1, Black women in the U.S. are three to four times more likely to die from pregnancy-related causes than white women (CDC, 2022).

These disparities are not due to biological differences, but to the cumulative impact of systemic racism, implicit bias, and discrimination in the healthcare system.

Implicit Bias

Implicit bias refers to the unconscious attitudes and stereotypes that affect our understanding, actions, and decisions. We all have implicit biases, shaped by our socialization and experiences.

In healthcare, implicit bias can lead to:

- **Differential Treatment:** Providers may treat BIPOC clients differently than white clients (e.g., spending less time with them, dismissing their concerns, providing less pain medication).

- **Stereotyping:** Providers may rely on stereotypes about BIPOC clients (e.g., assuming they are "strong" or have a high pain tolerance).
- **Miscommunication:** Providers may have difficulty communicating effectively with BIPOC clients due to cultural differences or language barriers.

Strategies for Providing Culturally Safe and Anti-Racist Care

Providing culturally safe and anti-racist care is an essential component of trauma-informed midwifery practice. It requires a commitment to ongoing learning, self-reflection, and systemic change.

Cultural Humility

Cultural humility is a lifelong process of self-reflection and self-critique, where we acknowledge our own biases and assumptions, and commit to learning from our clients about their cultural beliefs and practices (Tervalon & Murray-García, 1998).

Cultural humility is different from cultural competence, which often focuses on learning about the customs and traditions of different cultural groups. Cultural humility emphasizes the importance of recognizing and addressing power imbalances in the provider-client relationship.

Strategies for Practicing Cultural Humility

- **Self-Reflection:** Engage in ongoing self-reflection about your own biases, assumptions, and privileges.
- **Active Listening:** Listen actively and respectfully to your clients' experiences and perspectives.
- **Curiosity:** Be curious about your clients' cultural beliefs and practices, and ask open-ended questions to learn more.
- **Collaboration:** Collaborate with your clients to develop a plan of care that is respectful of their cultural values and preferences.
- **Accountability:** Take responsibility for your mistakes and commit to learning and growing.

Anti-Racism

Anti-racism is the active process of identifying and eliminating racism by changing systems, organizational structures, policies and practices and attitudes, so that power is redistributed and shared equitably (Comas-Díaz et al., 2019)

Strategies for Practicing Anti-Racist Care

- **Acknowledge Racism:** Acknowledge the reality of racism and its impact on the health and well-being of BIPOC clients.
- **Address Implicit Bias:** Actively work to identify and address your own implicit biases.
- **Challenge Discrimination:** Challenge racist remarks, behaviors, and policies in your workplace.
- **Advocate for Equity:** Advocate for policies and practices that promote racial equity in maternity care.
- **Center BIPOC Voices:** Center the voices and experiences of BIPOC clients and communities in your practice and advocacy efforts.

Caring for LGBTQIA+ Birthing People

LGBTQIA+ (Lesbian, Gay, Bisexual, Transgender, Queer, Intersex, Asexual) birthing people often face unique challenges and disparities in maternity care. They may experience discrimination, harassment, and lack of culturally competent care.

Understanding the Needs of LGBTQIA+ Birthing People

- **Trauma History:** LGBTQIA+ individuals have higher rates of trauma, including childhood abuse, sexual assault, and hate crimes.
- **Discrimination:** They may experience discrimination and mistreatment by healthcare providers due to their sexual orientation or gender identity.
- **Invisibility:** Their identities and families may be invisible or marginalized in the maternity care system.

- **Body Dysphoria:** Transgender and gender-nonconforming individuals may experience body dysphoria related to pregnancy and birth.

Strategies for Providing Gender-Affirming Care

- **Inclusive Language:** Use inclusive language that respects the diversity of gender identities and family structures (e.g., "birthing person" instead of "mother," "partner" instead of "husband").
- **Correct Names and Pronouns:** Ask clients what name and pronouns they use, and use them consistently.
- **Respect for Identity:** Respect the client's sexual orientation and gender identity without judgment or assumption.
- **Inclusive Forms and Policies:** Ensure that intake forms and policies are inclusive of LGBTQIA+ individuals and families.
- **Gender-Affirming Environment:** Create a welcoming and affirming environment (e.g., gender-neutral bathrooms, inclusive signage).
- **Trauma-Informed Approach:** Use a trauma-informed approach to care, recognizing the high rates of trauma in the LGBTQIA+ community.

Conclusion

Intersectionality, cultural humility, and anti-racism are essential components of trauma-informed midwifery care. By recognizing the impact of historical and systemic trauma, practicing cultural humility, and actively working to dismantle racism and oppression, we can create a maternity care system that is safe, equitable, and affirming for all birthing people.

In the next part of the book, we will explore the impact of trauma-informed care on the provider and the system, including strategies for preventing vicarious trauma and burnout, and implementing trauma-informed systems change.

Key Takeaways

- A trauma-informed approach must recognize the intersectionality of trauma with other identities and experiences.

- Historical trauma and racial trauma have a significant impact on the health and well-being of BIPOC birthing people.

- Racism and discrimination lead to significant disparities in maternal and infant health outcomes.

- Cultural humility is a lifelong process of self-reflection and self-critique that acknowledges and addresses power imbalances in the provider-client relationship.

- Anti-racism is the active process of identifying and eliminating racism in the maternity care system.

- LGBTQIA+ birthing people face unique challenges and require gender-affirming and trauma-informed care.

Chapter 14: Vicarious Trauma, Moral Injury, and Burnout

Working in midwifery is deeply rewarding, but it is also incredibly demanding. We witness the heights of human joy and the depths of human suffering. We hold space for trauma survivors, support families through crises, and navigate a broken healthcare system.

This work takes a toll. If we do not acknowledge and address the impact of this work on our own well-being, we risk experiencing vicarious trauma, moral injury, and burnout.

This chapter will explore these concepts and their impact on midwives. We will discuss strategies for recognizing the signs of secondary traumatic stress (STS) and compassion fatigue, and address the systemic factors that contribute to moral injury and burnout.

The Impact of Witnessing Traumatic Births

Witnessing traumatic births is a common experience for midwives. Whether the trauma is due to medical complications, obstetric violence, or the activation of the birthing person's past trauma, it can have a significant impact on the provider.

Secondary Traumatic Stress (STS)

Secondary traumatic stress (STS) is the emotional distress that results from hearing about the firsthand trauma experiences of another person (Figley, 1995). It is also known as *vicarious trauma*.

The symptoms of STS are similar to the symptoms of PTSD:

- **Intrusion:** Intrusive thoughts, images, or nightmares related to the traumatic births witnessed.
- **Avoidance:** Avoiding situations, people, or places that remind the provider of the trauma.

- **Negative Changes in Mood and Cognition:** Feeling cynical, hopeless, or numb; difficulty concentrating; negative beliefs about self or the world.
- **Hyperarousal:** Irritability, anxiety, hypervigilance, difficulty sleeping, exaggerated startle response.

Compassion Fatigue

Compassion fatigue is a broader term that encompasses both STS and burnout. It is the emotional and physical exhaustion that results from the chronic use of empathy when caring for others who are suffering (Figley, 1995).

Compassion fatigue can manifest as:

- **Emotional Numbness:** Feeling disconnected from emotions, difficulty empathizing with others.
- **Physical Exhaustion:** Chronic fatigue, headaches, digestive problems.
- **Loss of Meaning and Purpose:** Feeling disillusioned with the work, loss of sense of purpose.
- **Relationship Difficulties:** Difficulty connecting with family and friends.

Recognizing the Signs of STS and Compassion Fatigue

It is important to recognize the signs of STS and compassion fatigue early so you can take steps to address them.

Warning Signs:

- Dreading going to work.
- Feeling overwhelmed by the demands of the job.
- Difficulty sleeping or having nightmares.
- Increased irritability or anger.
- Feeling emotionally numb or detached.

- Increased use of alcohol or drugs to cope.
- Difficulty making decisions or concentrating.
- Physical symptoms (e.g., headaches, stomachaches).

Self-Assessment Tools

There are several self-assessment tools available to help you monitor your levels of STS and compassion fatigue, such as the Professional Quality of Life Scale (ProQOL) (Stamm, 2010).

Moral Injury When Systemic Constraints Prevent Quality Care

Moral injury is the psychological distress that results from actions, or the lack of action, which violate an individual's moral or ethical code (Shay, 2014). It occurs when individuals are forced to betray their own values and beliefs due to systemic constraints or organizational pressures.

In midwifery, moral injury can occur when:

- We are unable to provide the quality of care we believe our clients deserve due to staffing shortages, time constraints, or lack of resources.
- We are forced to implement policies or practices that we believe are harmful or unethical (e.g., coercive practices, disrespectful care).
- We witness obstetric violence or discrimination and are unable to intervene effectively.
- We feel unsupported by our organizations or leaders when we raise concerns about safety or quality of care.

The Impact of Moral Injury

Moral injury can lead to feelings of guilt, shame, anger, betrayal, and disillusionment. It can erode our sense of purpose and meaning in our work, and contribute to burnout and depression.

126

Addressing Moral Injury

Addressing moral injury requires recognizing that it is not an individual problem, but a systemic one. It requires organizational change and a commitment to creating a culture of ethical practice.

- **Acknowledge the Problem:** Acknowledge the reality of moral injury and its impact on providers.
- **Create a Culture of Safety:** Create a culture where providers feel safe to speak up about ethical concerns without fear of retaliation.
- **Promote Ethical Decision-Making:** Provide training and support for ethical decision-making in complex situations.
- **Advocate for Systemic Change:** Advocate for policies and practices that support ethical practice and quality care.

Burnout

Burnout is a state of emotional, physical, and mental exhaustion caused by excessive and prolonged stress. It is characterized by:

- **Exhaustion:** Feeling drained and depleted of energy.
- **Cynicism:** Feeling detached, negative, or cynical about the work.
- **Inefficacy:** Feeling incompetent or lacking accomplishment.

Factors Contributing to Burnout in Midwifery

- High workload and long hours.
- Staffing shortages.
- Lack of autonomy and control over the work environment.
- Exposure to trauma and suffering.
- Lack of support from colleagues and leaders.
- Bureaucratic constraints and paperwork burden.

Addressing Burnout

Addressing burnout requires a multi-faceted approach that includes individual coping strategies and organizational changes.

- **Individual Strategies:**
    - Prioritizing self-care (e.g., sleep, nutrition, exercise, mindfulness).
    - Setting boundaries and learning to say no.
    - Seeking support from colleagues, friends, and family.
    - Engaging in hobbies and activities outside of work.
- **Organizational Strategies:**
    - Improving staffing levels and reducing workload.
    - Promoting autonomy and shared governance.
    - Providing supportive leadership and supervision.
    - Creating a culture of appreciation and recognition.

Conclusion

Vicarious trauma, moral injury, and burnout are significant challenges for midwives. Recognizing the impact of this work on our well-being and taking proactive steps to address these issues are essential for sustaining a long and fulfilling career in midwifery.

In the next chapter, we will explore strategies for building resilience and promoting self-care for providers.

Key Takeaways

- Vicarious trauma (secondary traumatic stress) is the emotional distress that results from exposure to the trauma experiences of others.
- Compassion fatigue is the emotional and physical exhaustion that results from the chronic use of empathy when caring for others who are suffering.

- Moral injury is the psychological distress that results from violating one's moral or ethical code due to systemic constraints.

- Burnout is a state of emotional, physical, and mental exhaustion caused by excessive and prolonged stress.

- Recognizing the signs of STS, compassion fatigue, moral injury, and burnout is the first step toward addressing them.

- Addressing these issues requires a multi-faceted approach that includes individual coping strategies and organizational changes.

Chapter 15: Self-Care for Providers and Building Resilience

We cannot provide trauma-informed care if we are overwhelmed, dysregulated, and burned out. Our ability to be present, compassionate, and effective depends on our own well-being.

Self-care is not a luxury; it is an ethical imperative. It is the foundation of sustainable midwifery practice.

This chapter will explore evidence-based strategies for building resilience and promoting self-care for providers, including nervous system regulation, mindfulness, clinical supervision, and reflective practice. We will also discuss the organizational responsibility for provider well-being.

Evidence-Based Strategies for Provider Resilience

Resilience is the ability to bounce back from adversity and cope with stress in a healthy way. It is not something you are born with; it is a skill that can be developed and strengthened over time.

Nervous System Regulation

As we discussed in Chapter 2, the nervous system plays a crucial role in our response to stress. When we are chronically stressed, our nervous system can become dysregulated, leading to hyperarousal (anxiety, irritability) or hypoarousal (numbness, fatigue).

Nervous system regulation involves learning how to calm the nervous system and return to a state of balance (the window of tolerance).

Strategies for Nervous System Regulation:

- **Deep Breathing:** Slow, deep breathing activates the parasympathetic nervous system (the "brake") and promotes relaxation.

- **Grounding Techniques:** Grounding techniques (as discussed in Chapter 10) can help bring you back to the present moment and reconnect with your body.
- **Movement:** Physical activity, such as walking, yoga, dancing, or stretching, can help release stress hormones and regulate the nervous system.
- **Co-regulation:** Connecting with others who are calm and regulated can help calm your own nervous system.

Mindfulness

Mindfulness is the practice of paying attention to the present moment, on purpose, and without judgment. Mindfulness can help reduce stress, improve emotional regulation, and enhance compassion and empathy.

Strategies for Practicing Mindfulness:

- **Meditation:** Formal meditation practices, such as sitting meditation or walking meditation, can help train the mind to be more present and aware.
- **Informal Mindfulness:** Integrating mindfulness into daily activities, such as washing your hands, drinking coffee, or walking to work.
- **Self-Compassion:** Treating yourself with kindness, understanding, and acceptance, especially during difficult times.

Building a Self-Care Toolkit

Self-care looks different for everyone. It is important to develop a personalized self-care toolkit that includes strategies that work for you.

Categories of Self-Care:

- **Physical:** Sleep, nutrition, exercise, rest, healthcare.
- **Emotional:** Therapy, journaling, creative expression, connecting with emotions.
- **Social:** Connecting with friends and family, setting boundaries, asking for help.

- **Spiritual:** Connecting with nature, practicing gratitude, engaging in spiritual practices (if applicable).
- **Professional:** Clinical supervision, peer support, professional development, setting boundaries at work.

The Importance of Clinical Supervision and Reflective Practice

Clinical supervision and reflective practice are essential for promoting provider well-being and preventing burnout. They provide a safe space to process difficult experiences, explore ethical dilemmas, and enhance clinical skills.

Clinical Supervision

Clinical supervision is a formal relationship between a supervisor and a supervisee that focuses on the supervisee's professional development and well-being.

Benefits of Clinical Supervision:

- **Emotional Support:** A safe space to process emotions and receive support.
- **Skill Development:** Opportunities to enhance clinical skills and knowledge.
- **Ethical Guidance:** Guidance on navigating ethical dilemmas and challenges.
- **Reduced Burnout:** Reduced risk of burnout and compassion fatigue.

Reflective Practice

Reflective practice is the process of critically examining one's own experiences and actions to learn and grow.

Strategies for Reflective Practice:

- **Journaling:** Writing about your experiences and reflections.

- **Peer Supervision:** Meeting with colleagues to discuss cases and share perspectives.
- **Debriefing:** Debriefing difficult experiences with a trusted colleague or supervisor.
- **Mindfulness:** Paying attention to your thoughts, feelings, and actions in the moment.

Organizational Responsibility for Provider Well-being

While individual self-care strategies are important, they are not enough to address the systemic factors that contribute to burnout and moral injury. Organizations have a responsibility to create a culture that supports provider well-being and promotes ethical practice.

Strategies for Organizational Change:

- **Adequate Staffing:** Ensuring adequate staffing levels to manage workload and prevent burnout.
- **Supportive Leadership:** Providing supportive leadership that values provider well-being and promotes a culture of safety and respect.
- **Access to Resources:** Providing access to resources for mental health support, clinical supervision, and professional development.
- **Trauma-Informed Policies:** Implementing policies and practices that are trauma-informed for both clients and staff.
- **Recognition and Appreciation:** Recognizing and appreciating the contributions of staff.

Conclusion

Self-care and resilience are essential for sustainable midwifery practice. By prioritizing our own well-being, we can enhance our capacity to provide compassionate and effective care to our clients. However, individual self-care is not enough. We must also advocate for organizational changes that support provider well-being and promote a culture of ethical practice.

In the final chapter of this book, we will explore strategies for implementing trauma-informed systems change in maternity care.

Key Takeaways

- Self-care is an ethical imperative for midwives.
- Resilience is a skill that can be developed and strengthened over time.
- Nervous system regulation strategies (e.g., deep breathing, grounding, movement) can help manage stress and promote balance.
- Mindfulness practices can reduce stress, improve emotional regulation, and enhance compassion.
- Clinical supervision and reflective practice are essential for promoting provider well-being and preventing burnout.
- Organizations have a responsibility to create a culture that supports provider well-being and promotes ethical practice.

Chapter 16: Implementing Trauma-Informed Systems

Trauma-informed care is not just about individual practices; it is about systemic change. To truly create a maternity care system that is safe, supportive of agency, and healing, we must implement trauma-informed principles at all levels of the system, from policy to practice.

This chapter will explore strategies for creating change at the practice or hospital level, discuss policy recommendations and advocacy efforts, and envision the future of trauma-informed midwifery education.

Creating Change at the Practice or Hospital Level

Implementing trauma-informed systems change requires a comprehensive approach that involves organizational commitment, staff training, policy revision, environmental modifications, and ongoing evaluation.

The Implementation Process

The implementation of trauma-informed care is a process that unfolds over time. It typically involves the following stages:

1. **Awareness and Commitment:** Raising awareness about the impact of trauma and securing commitment from leadership and staff to implement trauma-informed care.
2. **Assessment and Planning:** Conducting an assessment of the organization's current practices and developing a plan for implementation.
3. **Training and Education:** Providing training and education to all staff on the principles and practices of trauma-informed care.
4. **Policy and Practice Change:** Revising policies and practices to align with trauma-informed principles.
5. **Environmental Modifications:** Modifying the physical environment to promote safety and comfort.

6. **Evaluation and Sustainability:** Evaluating the impact of the implementation efforts and developing strategies for sustainability.

Key Strategies for Implementation

- **Leadership Engagement:** Engage leadership at all levels of the organization to champion the implementation efforts.
- **Staff Involvement:** Involve staff at all levels of the organization in the planning and implementation process.
- **Client Involvement:** Involve clients and community members in the implementation process to ensure that the changes are responsive to their needs.
- **Trauma-Informed Champions:** Identify and support trauma-informed champions within the organization who can lead the implementation efforts.
- **Pilot Projects:** Start with small pilot projects to test and refine the implementation strategies before scaling up.
- **Ongoing Support:** Provide ongoing support and coaching to staff as they implement the changes.

Policy Recommendations and Advocacy

Policy change is essential for creating a trauma-informed maternity care system. We must advocate for policies that support the principles of trauma-informed care and promote equity and justice in maternity care.

Policy Recommendations

- **Reimbursement for Trauma-Informed Care:** Advocate for reimbursement models that support the provision of trauma-informed care, including longer appointment times, continuity of care models, and trauma-specific screening and treatment.
- **Workforce Development:** Advocate for policies that support the development of a diverse and trauma-informed midwifery workforce, including funding for training and education, loan repayment programs, and equitable reimbursement rates.

- **Anti-Racism and Equity:** Advocate for policies that address racism and discrimination in maternity care and promote racial equity in maternal and infant health outcomes.
- **Paid Family Leave:** Advocate for paid family leave policies that support the well-being of birthing people and their families during the postpartum period.
- **Access to Mental Health Services:** Advocate for policies that improve access to affordable and culturally responsive mental health services for perinatal populations.

Advocacy Efforts

Midwives can play a crucial role in advocating for policy change at the local, state, and national levels.

- **Professional Organizations:** Engage with professional organizations (e.g., ACNM, MANA) to advocate for trauma-informed policies and practices.
- **Legislative Advocacy:** Contact legislators and policymakers to educate them about the importance of trauma-informed care and advocate for specific policy changes.
- **Community Organizing:** Collaborate with community organizations and advocacy groups to advocate for systemic change in maternity care.
- **Research and Data Collection:** Conduct research and collect data on the impact of trauma and the effectiveness of trauma-informed care to inform policy and practice.

The Future of Trauma-Informed Midwifery Education

To create a trauma-informed maternity care system, we must transform how we educate and train midwives. Trauma-informed principles must be integrated into all aspects of midwifery education, from the curriculum to the clinical training.

Curriculum Integration

- **Comprehensive Trauma Education:** Integrate comprehensive education on the prevalence, impact, and neurobiology of trauma into the midwifery curriculum.
- **Trauma-Informed Skills Training:** Provide training on trauma-informed communication, assessment, and intervention skills.
- **Anti-Racism and Cultural Humility:** Integrate education on anti-racism, cultural humility, and systemic trauma into the curriculum.
- **Interprofessional Education:** Provide opportunities for interprofessional education with other healthcare professionals (e.g., nurses, physicians, social workers) on trauma-informed care.

Clinical Training

- **Trauma-Informed Preceptorship:** Provide clinical training in settings that model trauma-informed care and offer mentorship by trauma-informed preceptors.
- **Reflective Practice:** Integrate reflective practice and clinical supervision into the clinical training to support students in processing difficult experiences and developing resilience.
- **Simulation:** Use simulation training to practice trauma-informed skills in a safe and supportive environment.

A Vision for the Future

The vision for the future of trauma-informed midwifery care is a system where every birthing person feels safe, respected, and supported in their agency. It is a system where the impact of trauma is recognized and addressed, and where healing and resilience are promoted.

This vision requires a collective effort from midwives, educators, researchers, policymakers, and community members. It requires a commitment to ongoing learning, self-reflection, and systemic change.

The path toward a trauma-informed maternity care system is long and challenging, but it is essential for the health and well-being of birthing people, families, and communities.

Final Thoughts

Trauma-informed care is not just a buzzword or a trend. It is a fundamental shift in how we approach healthcare. It is a recognition of the significant impact of trauma on the lives of the people we care for, and a commitment to providing care that is safe, compassionate, and healing.

As midwives, we are uniquely positioned to lead this transformation in maternity care. We have the skills, the knowledge, and the passion to create a system where every birth is a positive and supportive experience.

The work is hard, but the rewards are immense. When we practice trauma-informed care, we not only improve health outcomes, but we also support the healing and resilience of the human spirit.

Key Takeaways

- Implementing trauma-informed care requires systemic change at all levels of the system, from policy to practice.

- Creating change at the practice or hospital level involves organizational commitment, staff training, policy revision, and environmental modifications.

- Policy recommendations include reimbursement for trauma-informed care, workforce development, anti-racism and equity, paid family leave, and access to mental health services.

- Midwives can play a crucial role in advocating for policy change through professional organizations, legislative advocacy, and community organizing.

- The future of trauma-informed midwifery education requires integrating trauma-informed principles into all aspects of the curriculum and clinical training.
- The vision for the future is a maternity care system where every birthing person feels safe, respected, and supported in their agency.

Appendices

A: Key Assessment and Screening Tools (Printable formats)

- Adverse Childhood Experiences (ACEs) Questionnaire
- PTSD Checklist for DSM-5 (PCL-5)
- Perinatal PTSD Questionnaire (PPQ)

B: Checklist for a Trauma-Informed Environment

Waiting Room:

- Is the lighting soft and warm?
- Is the noise level minimized?
- Is the furniture comfortable and accommodating for different body sizes?
- Are there clear pathways and exits?
- Is the signage inclusive and welcoming?

Exam Rooms:

- Are there dimmer switches on the overhead lights?
- Are there lamps with soft, warm bulbs?
- Is the room private and secure?
- Is the furniture arranged to promote collaboration and minimize power differentials?
- Are there resources available for grounding and coping (e.g., stress balls, aromatherapy)?

Staff Interactions:

- Do staff greet clients warmly and introduce themselves clearly?
- Do staff speak in a calm, respectful tone of voice?

- Do staff ask for permission before touching clients?
- Do staff respect clients' privacy and confidentiality?

C: Sample Scripts for Sensitive Conversations and Consent

Asking about Trauma History:

"Because experiences in our past can affect our health and well-being, we ask all of our clients about things like violence, abuse, and trauma. Is it okay if I ask you a few questions about your experiences? You don't have to answer any questions you don't want to."

Responding to Disclosure of Trauma:

"Thank you for sharing that with me. I know it can be difficult to talk about. I'm so sorry that happened to you. It makes sense that you would feel [scared/angry/anxious] given what you've been through. I want you to know that you are not alone, and help is available."

Obtaining Informed Consent:

"I'd like to talk to you about [procedure/treatment]. Here are the benefits, risks, and alternatives. What are your thoughts? What is most important to you? Do you consent to this plan?"

Trauma-Informed Cervical Check:

"I'd like to offer a cervical check now to see how your labor is progressing. It involves me inserting two fingers into your vagina to feel your cervix. Are you okay with that? We can go slowly, and if you want me to stop at any time, just say 'stop,' and I will immediately remove my hands."

D: Birth Plan Template for Trauma Survivors

My Birth Preferences

Name:

Due Date:

Support Persons:

My History:

(Optional: Share any history of trauma or abuse that you want your providers to know about.)

My Triggers:

(List any triggers that may cause you distress during labor and birth.)

My Coping Strategies:

(List any coping strategies that help you feel safe and grounded.)

Environment:

- Lighting (dim/bright):
- Sound (quiet/music):
- Privacy (minimal intrusions/visitors welcome):

Communication:

- How I prefer to be addressed:
- How I prefer to communicate my needs:
- Language preferences:

Consent:

- Please ask for explicit consent before touching me or performing any procedures.
- Please explain what you are doing and why before you do it.

Intimate Exams (Cervical Checks):

- Frequency (minimal/regular):
- Technique (gentle, slow, adequate lubrication):
- Positioning preferences:
- Stop signal:

Pain Management:

- Non-pharmacological preferences (movement, hydrotherapy, breathing techniques):
- Pharmacological preferences (nitrous oxide, epidural):
- Fears or concerns about pain management:

Interventions:

- Preferences regarding induction/augmentation:
- Preferences regarding fetal monitoring (intermittent/continuous):
- Preferences regarding episiotomy:

Pushing Stage:

- Positioning preferences (upright, side-lying):
- Pushing style (instinctive/coached):
- Exposure preferences:

Immediate Postpartum:

- Skin-to-skin contact (immediate/delayed):
- Cord clamping (delayed/immediate):
- Perineal repair (consent, anesthesia, support):

Infant Feeding:

- Feeding preferences (breastfeeding/chestfeeding, formula feeding):
- Support needs:

E: Grounding Techniques Handout

Grounding Techniques for Managing Stress and Anxiety

Grounding techniques can help you return to the present moment and reconnect with your body when you are feeling overwhelmed, anxious, or disconnected.

5-4-3-2-1 Technique:

- Identify 5 things you can see.
- Identify 4 things you can touch.
- Identify 3 things you can hear.
- Identify 2 things you can smell.
- Identify 1 thing you can taste.

Physical Grounding:

- Press your feet into the floor.
- Squeeze a stress ball or hold an object in your hand.
- Gently stretch or move your body.
- Notice the temperature of the air on your skin.

Breathing Techniques:

- Take slow, deep breaths. Breathe in through your nose and out through your mouth.
- Place a hand on your belly and feel it rise and fall with each breath.

Orienting to the Present:

- Remind yourself where you are and what day it is.
- Look around the room and notice the objects and colors.
- Listen to the sounds around you.

Temperature Change:

- Hold an ice cube in your hand.
- Splash cold water on your face.
- Drink a cold glass of water.

Movement:

- Rock or sway gently.
- Walk or pace slowly.
- Shake out your arms and legs.

F: Referral Resources (National and International)

United States:

- **National Domestic Violence Hotline:** 1-800-799-SAFE (7233) or text "START" to 88788
- **RAINN (Rape, Abuse & Incest National Network):** 1-800-656-HOPE (4673)
- **Postpartum Support International (PSI):** 1-800-944-4PPD (4773)
- **National Suicide Prevention Lifeline:** 988
- **The Trevor Project (LGBTQIA+ Suicide Prevention):** 1-866-488-7386 or text "START" to 678-678

Canada:

- **Ending Violence Association of Canada:** https://endingviolencecanada.org/getting-help-2/
- **Canadian Resource Centre for Victims of Crime:** 1-877-232-2610
- **Postpartum Support International (PSI) - Canada:** https://psidirectory.com/canada

United Kingdom:

- **National Domestic Abuse Helpline:** 0808 2000 247
- **Rape Crisis England & Wales:** 0808 802 9999
- **PANDAS Foundation (Perinatal Mental Health Support):** 0808 1961 776
- **Samaritans (Suicide Prevention):** 116 123

Australia:

- **1800RESPECT (Domestic, Family and Sexual Violence Counselling Service):** 1800 737 732
- **PANDA (Perinatal Anxiety & Depression Australia):** 1300 726 306
- **Lifeline (Suicide Prevention):** 13 11 14

International:

- **International Domestic Violence Resource Guide:** https://www.hotpeachpages.net/
- **International Directory of Rape Crisis Centers:** https://www.ibiblio.org/rcip/internl.html
- **Postpartum Support International (PSI) - International Directory:** https://psidirectory.com/

References

(1) Substance Abuse and Mental Health Services Administration. (2014). *SAMHSA's concept of trauma and guidance for a trauma-informed approach.* HHS Publication No. (SMA) 14-4884.

(2) Beck, C. T. (2004). Birth trauma: In the eye of the beholder. *Nursing Research, 53*(1), 28-35.

(3) Felitti, V. J., Anda, R. F., Nordenberg, D., Williamson, D. F., Spitz, A. M., Edwards, V., ... & Marks, J. S. (1998). Relationship of childhood abuse and household dysfunction to many of the leading causes of adult death. The Adverse Childhood Experiences (ACE) Study. *American Journal of Preventive Medicine, 14*(4), 245-258.

(4) Creedy, D. K., Shochet, I. M., & Horsfall, J. (2000). Childbirth and the development of acute trauma symptoms: incidence and contributing factors. *Birth, 27*(2), 104-111.

(5) Harris, R., & Ayers, S. (2012). What makes labour and birth traumatic? A survey of intrapartum 'hotspots'. *Psychology & Health, 27*(10), 1166-1177.

(6) Yildiz, P. D., Ayers, S., & Phillips, L. (2017). The prevalence of posttraumatic stress disorder in pregnancy and after birth: A systematic review and meta-analysis. *Journal of Affective Disorders, 208*, 634-645.

(7) Black, M. C., Basile, K. C., Breiding, M. J., Smith, S. G., Walters, M. L., Merrick, M. T., ... & Stevens, M. R. (2011). *The National Intimate Partner and Sexual Violence Survey (NISVS): 2010 summary report.* National Center for Injury Prevention and Control, Centers for Disease Control and Prevention.

(8) Silverman, J. G., Decker, M. R., Reed, E., & Raj, A. (2006). Intimate partner violence victimization before and during pregnancy among women residing in 26 US states: associations with maternal and

neonatal health. *American Journal of Obstetrics and Gynecology,* *195*(1), 140-148.

(9) Comas-Díaz, L. (2016). Racial trauma recovery: A race-informed therapeutic approach to racial wounds. In A. N. Alvarez, C. T. H. Liang, & H. A. Neville (Eds.), *The cost of racism for people of color: Contextualizing experiences of discrimination* (pp. 249–272). American Psychological Association.

(10) Centers for Disease Control and Prevention. (2020). *Pregnancy-related deaths.*

(11) Yehuda, R., & Lehrner, A. (2018). Intergenerational transmission of trauma effects: putative role of epigenetic mechanisms. *World Psychiatry, 17*(3), 243-257.

(12) Beck, C. T., & Watson, S. (2008). Impact of birth trauma on breast-feeding: a tale of two pathways. *Nursing Research, 57*(4), 228-236.

(13) Kendall-Tackett, K. A. (2007). A new paradigm for depression in new mothers: the central role of inflammation and how breastfeeding and anti-inflammatory treatments protect maternal mental health. *International Breastfeeding Journal, 2*(1), 1-14.

(14) Ayers, S., Bond, R., Bertullies, S., & Wijma, K. (2016). The aetiology of post-traumatic stress following childbirth: a meta-analysis and theoretical framework. *Psychological Medicine, 46*(6), 1121-1134.

(15) Van der Kolk, B. A. (2014). *The body keeps the score: Brain, mind, and body in the healing of trauma.* Viking.

(16) Porges, S. W. (2011). *The polyvagal theory: Neurophysiological foundations of emotions, attachment, communication, and self-regulation.* W. W. Norton & Company.

(17) Walker, P. (2013). *Complex PTSD: From surviving to thriving: A guide and map for recovering from childhood trauma.* CreateSpace Independent Publishing Platform.

(18) Buckley, S. J. (2015). *Hormonal physiology of childbearing: Evidence and implications for women, babies, and healthcare.* Childbirth Connection.

(19) Dick-Read, G. (1944). *Childbirth without fear: The principles and practice of natural childbirth.* Heinemann Medical Books.

(20) Siegel, D. J. (1999). *The developing mind: Toward a neurobiology of interpersonal experience.* Guilford Press.

(21) Tervalon, M., & Murray-García, J. (1998). Cultural humility versus cultural competence: a critical distinction in defining physician training outcomes in multicultural education. Journal of health care for the poor and underserved, 9(2), 117-125.

(22) Weathers, F.W., Litz, B.T., Keane, T.M., Palmieri, P.A., Marx, B.P., & Schnurr, P.P. (2013). The PTSD Checklist for DSM-5 (PCL-5). Scale available from the National Center for PTSD at www.ptsd.va.gov.

(23) Callahan, J. L., Borja, S. E., & Hynan, L. S. (2006). Development and validation of the Perinatal Posttraumatic Stress Disorder Questionnaire. Journal of Traumatic Stress, 19(1), 117-126.

(24) Elwyn, G., Frosch, D. L., Thomson, R., Joseph-Williams, N., Lloyd, A., Kinnersley, P., ... & Barry, M. J. (2017). Shared decision making: a model for clinical practice. Journal of general internal medicine, 32(10), 1361-1367.

(25) Sandall, J., Soltani, H., Gates, S., Shennan, A., & Devane, D. (2016). Midwife-led continuity models versus other models of care for childbearing women. Cochrane Database of Systematic Reviews, (4).

(26) Grekin, R., & O'Hara, M. W. (2014). Prevalence and risk factors of postpartum posttraumatic stress disorder: a meta-analysis. Clinical psychology review, 34(5), 389-401. [Repeat of Ref 9]

(27) Geronimus, A. T., Hicken, M., Keene, D., & Bound, J. (2006). "Weathering" and age patterns of allostatic load scores among blacks and whites in the United States. American journal of public health, 96(5), 826-833.

Comas-Díaz, L., Nagayama Hall, G., Neville, H. A., & Kazak, A. E. (Eds.). (2019). Racial trauma: Theory, research, and healing [Special issue]. American Psychologist, 74(1).

(29) Centers for Disease Control and Prevention (CDC). (2022). Racial/Ethnic Disparities in Pregnancy-Related Deaths. [Repeat of Ref 10, updated year]